Also by Andrew Duxbury...

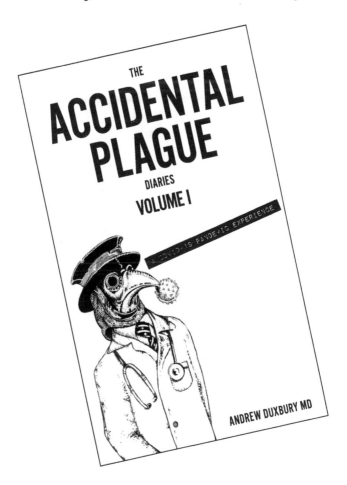

Winner – Gold Medal – Independent Publishers Book Awards

Winner – Gold Medal – Nonfiction Authors Association

Winner – Bronze Medal – Reader Views Literary Awards

Finalist – Next Generation Indie Book Awards

Finalist – Eric Hoffer Book Awards – Grand Prize and Montaigne Medal

The Accidental Plague Diaries
Volume II

❧

COVID-19 Variants and Vaccinations

For Dee —

In gratitude this translation
for your work with southern
Queen Whitlers.

[signature]

THE

ACCIDENTAL
PLAGUE

DIARIES

VOLUME II

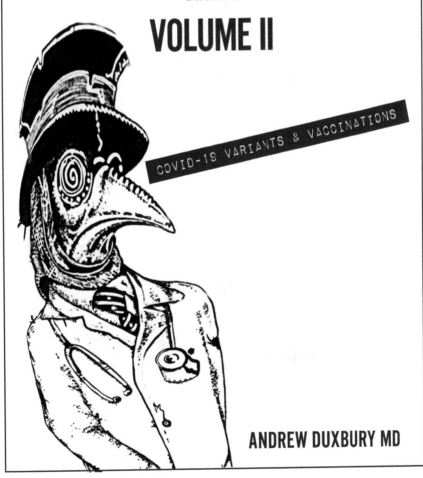

COVID-19 VARIANTS & VACCINATIONS

ANDREW DUXBURY MD

The Accidental Plague Diaries, Volume II: COVID-19 Variants and Vaccinations

Development Editing by Steve Peha
Layout and Design by Steve Peha
Cover Illustration by Jeannie Duxbury

Printed in the United States of America.

Published by:

Singular Books
An Imprint of Platform Publishing
543 NE 84th St.
Seattle, WA 98115

ISBN: 978-0-9972831-8-1

For Craig and Vickie.

Here's to us! Who's like us? Damned few...

ACKNOWLEDGMENTS

ONCE AGAIN I MUST CONFESS that no volume of prose appears due to the labors of a single author. I continue to owe a huge debt of gratitude to Steve Peha, my editor and publisher, and the man behind Singular Books who shepherded my original essays into a highly readable and award-winning book. He continues to spin gold from the straw of my words, often written late at night in a rather slapdash fashion, making me sound far less confused than I actually am by the weighty subjects I tackle in these writings.

My sister, Jeannie Duxbury Rae, has once again graciously picked up her pen and lent her talents to both cover and interior art.

But my biggest debt of gratitude is reserved for my friends, my patients, and various random strangers who have continued to read my COVID writings, given me the positive feedback, in writing and in person, that has allowed me to continue to think and analyze this peculiar moment in American and world history, and made sure that there is meaning and purpose in *The Accidental Plague Diaries* beyond my personal brand of navel-gazing.

TABLE OF CONTENTS

I often reflected upon the unprovided condition that the whole body of the people were in at the first coming of this calamity upon them, and how it was for want of timely entering into measures and managements, as well public as private, that all the confusions that followed were brought upon us, and that such a prodigious number of people sank in that disaster, which, if proper steps had been taken, might, Providence concurring, have been avoided, and which, if posterity think fit, they may take a caution and warning from.—Dainiel DeFoe, *A Journal of the Plague Year*

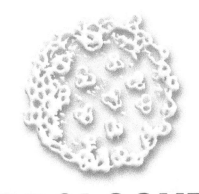

PROLOGUE
*Where Is the Life
That Late I Led?*

This is the text of the remarks I delivered from the pulpit of the Unitarian Universalist Church of Birmingham on Sunday, December 5, 2021.

WHEN REVEREND JULIE ASKED ME if I would do a Sunday in the pulpit for her during her time away, I immediately said yes. One does not cross Reverend Julie.

She asked me if I could base it in some way around my recent writing, so I immediately came up with a catchy title: *Book Writing and Other Happy Accidents.* I then promptly forgot about the commitment until a couple of weeks ago when I realized that the date I had agreed to was rapidly approaching and that I had better get something down on paper so as not to look like a total fool up here.

This is not the first time I've stood before you. That was August 5, 2001. You might ask how I remember the date so exactly. It was four days after the death of Steve, my first husband. I had agreed a few weeks prior to give a talk from the pulpit about aging, using a lot of the materials I use in my teaching of older patients and their families.

Even though I was grieving and suffering from a significant loss, I decided the best thing for me psychologically was to get up there and keep moving and keep living. I was 39 years old. I had been with Steve for 13 years. I recognized that even though his life was over, mine was not, and that I had better begin the process of figuring out a life that no longer included him.

Those of you who have been around for a while might remember Steve. You never got to see him in his full robust health, but even in his diminished energy, as his disease slowly turned his lungs into hunks of useless, fibrotic tissue, he was a force of nature.

He had a huge impact on our new friends in Birmingham, where we had only been for a short time. His wit, his impish humor, his artistic talents—they all made an impression.

Steve had originally come out as gay at the age of 14 in 1962, a time when such things just weren't done. He fought his entire adult life to be recognized as a unique and valuable human being against a society that spent most of its time trying to silence him. But he wasn't about to let that happen.

When we met in 1989, he was 40 years old. He'd been through the fire of the AIDS crisis in the LA area over the previous decade, losing most of his close friends. His relocation to Northern California to take care of his terminally ill mother, which ended up bringing us together, had him determined to live a different, more coherent life. I ended up being the one with whom he built it. He may have been 14 years my senior, but I was the mature one.

His death left an enormous void, and it did a couple of things that ended up impacting my life in enormous ways. I didn't plan them. They became happy accidents of the type that have guided my life over the decades.

The first was that it allowed me to begin separating my personal identity from that of my professional career as a physician. This process had begun several years before, but Steve's illness and needs over his last few years greatly accelerated it.

I set foot on an educational treadmill at the age of four when I first headed off to pre-school three days a week. Preschool led to kindergarten (where I was a challenge as I could already read; I was a precocious little twerp) which led to elementary school which led to middle school (best forgotten) which led to high school which led to college (two majors; one wasn't enough) which led to medical school which led to residency which led to fellowship which led to faculty appointment.

At this time, I was trying to play the game of working my way up the academic ladder to a deanship or some such by balancing research with a clinical career. However, I ran afoul of politics in the University of California system in the late 90s—a miserable experience at the time, but it ended up being yet another happy accident as it required a swift relocation to UAB due to my need for a steady paycheck.

I was hopeful this Deep South adventure (I had never set foot in the state of Alabama until I came for my initial interview) would last for no more than four or five years, but Steve's illness manifested roughly a year after our arrival.

He needed me at home, and he needed my energy. Something had to give.

What gave was my ability to play the games needed to move forward academically or with a research agenda. I settled into a purely clinical/education role where I had more control over my schedule.

Another happy accident manifested after he was gone: I found myself with unstructured time and energy and no real idea what to do with it all.

Unitarian Universalist Church of Birmingham to the rescue.

The congregation stuck me on the board under the presidency of a local actress and drama teacher. I didn't know her well but knew she had grown up in the church and was an important part of how everything functioned.

At my first board meeting, I was tired. I kicked off my shoes. Put my feet up and asked, "What now?" Our esteemed board president took one look at me, twiddling my socked toes in a board meeting, and decided I was her kind of person. We remain fast friends and co-conspirators to this day.

The first thing she asked me to do was to help put together entertainment for the Stewardship dinner. So, in the fall of 2002, I found myself hauling out my very rusty theatrical skills. I had been a stage manager, director, and all-around techie for theater in my teens and early 20s but had given it all up when I hit residency. Every third night on call and theater simply don't go together.

She asked me if I might want to perform, and together we cooked up a vaudeville in which I played a figure derived from the Emcee from the musical Cabaret. She played a variant on Marlene Dietrich. We didn't know it at the time, but the first seeds of the *Politically Incorrect Cabaret* had been sown.

A few days before the one and only show, I accepted a blind date with a guy I'd been chatting with online. His name was Tommy. Over the next few weeks, we ran into each other in a number of contexts.

He had attended the Unitarian Church in the past and had decided to come back. He was given my name as a resource for aging programs he was developing at his job. He was the chief nursing officer for Birmingham Healthcare at the time.

After the third time we ran into each other, I decided the universe was trying to tell me something, so we went out again. And again. And ten months later he moved in. Our relationship was another happy accident.

I had been dating a series of highly inappropriate men over the course of the previous year and had pretty much concluded that I needed to swear off dating and romantic entanglements. So I spent the first six months of our dating life trying to figure out how to politely dump him as I knew that a second relationship was just never going to succeed. Fortunately, even I was eventually able to see that what we had was working, so I gave up on that plan.

Tommy's and my courtship was held in full view of the Unitarian Church and its congregation. It quickly received a stamp of approval from various sources including the then Reverend, and various senior congregants who had been worried that I might turn into a recluse or, worse yet, move back to the West Coast.

I was thinking seriously about it.

I had been interviewing for jobs in California, Oregon, and Washington. None of them had panned out. Some were not a good fit for my skill set. A couple didn't like the fact that I was an openly gay man. One strung me along for some months, using me as a motivator to get an internal candidate to say yes and sign a contract.

Eventually, UAB figured out I was looking and, not wanting to lose me, cast around for something that would nail my feet to the floor for a while. Another happy accident: a wealthy donor decided just at that time to endow the clinical geriatrics program with a sum of money that would allow me to redesign the geriatrics clinic from the ground up in my image and to my specifications. I wasn't going to get anything better than that on the West Coast, so the job hunt ended.

><

Tommy and I were now a stable couple and work had new purpose, but I still found myself with excess time and energy. Tommy, having always been involved in the performing arts as a classical musician, suggested we go through the door that my church family had opened, and that we start getting involved in the local music theater scene. So we did.

I found that I was actually not untalented, as I had long believed, and Tommy started to slide from performance into more production roles like stage management, wardrobe, and, of course, wigs—yet another happy accident.

I was playing the mayor in *The Best Little Whorehouse in Texas* at the Virginia Samford Theater and Tommy was hanging around backstage one night during tech rehearsal. A good friend of ours was costuming and also appearing on stage and was getting frazzled as there was too much for her to do.

She looked at Tommy and asked him if he could do finger waves in a set of 1930s period wigs for the opening number. His response was "I don't know. Show me." She did, and he plunged his hands into a bunch of acrylic hair and realized he really enjoyed working with it.

He approached his wig work as sculpture, just using highly unusual materials, and it didn't take long before he was the go-to person for theatrical wigs in Birmingham. I would never have predicted a full wig studio as part of my home.

For 15 years, happy accident followed happy accident.

A major downturn in Tommy's work life as a nurse executive led to his returning to school to get the music degree he had always wanted. Production problems at Opera Birmingham which we were able to solve led to my ending up in the opera chorus and Tommy as the managing director.

We became fixtures in the performing arts community of Birmingham. We hadn't intended for it to be that way. It just happened as one thing led to another. We thought it would go on like that for decades. It didn't.

As most of you know, in the spring of 2018, Tommy became rapidly ill with previously unrecognized heart disease. He died suddenly in the hospital of complications from his treatment.

I'd been through this widowhood thing before and thought I could handle it. What I hadn't counted on was how much remained unresolved from my first widowhood 17 years before. I also came to the realization that widowhood at 39 and widowhood at 56 are somewhat different.

At 39, you know you're still young and that you have a life spread out before you, even as a gay man, where 39 is considered four years dead and buried.

56 is different. You're looking more at retirement rushing down on you rather than at decades of career and life building. I wasn't sure

what to do or how to handle things.

In those first few months when I was starting to take stock of my life and figure out what should come next, I had to come to grips with the fact that I was very definitely an elder, especially in the gay community. Those in my peer group were starting to become grandparents. People were starting to discuss investments and retirement portfolios at parties.

I had to face up to the fact that, without ever having bothered to have children, I was a *paw paw*. I've made a professional study of aging for decades. I know a lot about it, and I've seen the psychological adjustments that older adults have to make. I realized I needed to make some of those for myself.

One of the things I have learned is that it is the natural and proper role of the elder to be the storyteller, the keeper of culture and of wisdom. I had any number of stories from my life and now no one to share them with, so I started to write them down.

I had written a few long posts on Facebook to update friends on Tommy's illness and death, so I kept them up. I wrote about my day. I wrote anecdotes about my and Tommy's and Steve's lives. I wrote my reactions to politics and social trends.

Obviously, I had not taken the lessons of Ginny Weasley and diaries that write back at you to heart. People started to read these posts, to comment, and to encourage my writing. So I kept at it.

The posts eventually became a blog. It had no specific intent. It was just one confused and lonely man trying to make sense of a muddle.

In the early winter of 2020, I had been writing for about a year and a half. I was concentrating mainly on work and on what I was up to theatrically. There were whispers in the media about a new and rapidly spreading coronavirus half a world away, but I was naïve enough to assume that the agencies of the federal government designed to protect public health would swing into play, and life would go on. It didn't.

I was pretty sure I knew where we were heading in late February, but I didn't want to write about the epidemic that was rapidly moving towards a pandemic. Writing about it would make it real, something I would have to face and grapple with head-on.

Finally, on March 10, 2020, the day before the World Health Organization declared the coronavirus a pandemic, I sat down and wrote the following:

I am a doctor. It is time to make sense of my existential angst. My brothers and sisters in healthcare professions are feeling it. We're all watching a viral pandemic unroll in real-time right in front of us. We all know far too much about the ramifications of where the coronavirus may lead.

This was the first paragraph of the first entry in what I would end up calling *The Accidental Plague Diaries*.

Once the flood gates were opened, I began to write about the coronavirus frequently and in-depth, trying to parse out the narrative of what was happening to our society and to make sure that I understood the trends—societal and scientific—properly.

After about a month, I looked back on what I had written and realized I was writing a plague diary. It's a literary form that's been around for millennia. It's usually written by a private citizen chronicling what happens to their society under the pressures of pandemic illness.

Plague diaries become valuable tools in understanding the social impact of disease, concentrating on the more mundane aspects of daily living that are often left out of government reports and chronicles.

I hadn't intended to do this; it was an accident.

I received a good deal of feedback from people thanking me for my writings as they seemed to help them make sense of the pandemic and societal changes in reaction thereto. There's nothing like having someone say they like your writing to get you to write some more. So I kept on.

By midsummer, I looked back at what I had written and started to wonder if what I was writing was something more than Facebook or blog posts. Was my *Accidental Plague Diary* something that might be helpful and of interest to those outside my immediate circle of acquaintance?

I contacted an old friend, whom I have known since elementary school, who is in the micro-publishing business. I sent him what I had written so far and asked him what he thought. He thought it was a book and that he would be publishing it. I kept writing.

How did I learn to write? I did have an expensive formal education which included a top-ranked prep school and Stanford University, but I don't think they were really responsible. They gave me a background in grammar and an ability to be a decent technical writer, but that's not really my forté.

Again, another happy accident, this one involving genetics.

I have told my patients for years that the most important thing one can do to age successfully is to choose their parents carefully. I lucked out with my mother. The daughter of British emigrés, she had a love of language and words and taught me more about a well-turned phrase than any professor I ever had.

And then there was Stephen Sondheim.

To me, a musical theater nerd coming of age in the late 70s and early 80s, he was Shakespeare. His ability to choose exactly the right word to form a lyric that would both cut you with its emotion and shock you with its cleverness played right into my personality.

I've tried for years to even begin to do what he did seemingly so effortlessly. I don't think I've ever succeeded although he did call a piece of mine that a mutual friend sent to him "Brilliant!"—so there is that. Thank god he lived long enough for me to be able to send him a copy of the first volume of this book. Its chapter titles are an homage.

><•0

At the end of last year, my publisher and I decided we had a fully formed book that merely required editing. It wasn't a book I had intended to write. It was yet another happy accident.

I kept the *Accidental Plague Diaries* as a title because I'd gotten used to it. I pluralized it deliberately. Both because the book was written accidentally and also because the plague itself was accidental. If it had hit at a different time in history with a different administration in power, it would likely not have taken the same form that it did.

Will there be another? A Volume 2? *The Accidental Plague Diaries 2 – Delta Dawn? The Accidental Plague Diaries 2 – Electric Deltaloo?* I don't know. The material is written in blog form. It could easily be converted to another book. I just don't want to repeat myself or bore my audience. I figure I'll wait until something happens in the next couple of months and the next happy accident ricochets my life in a way that will let me know what's next.

Thank you.

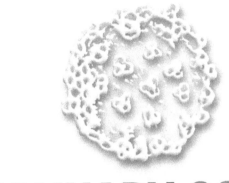

JANUARY 2021

It All Seems So Long Ago

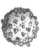

SATURDAY | JANUARY 23, 2021

SOMETHING SEEMS TO HAVE HAPPENED to my perception of time.

It feels normal in the immediate here and now, but once something slips into the past, it's as if there's a great acceleration. Perhaps it's the dizzying pace of events as the country reels from political and public health upheavals. Perhaps this is what happens when we age.

My patients have always talked about time moving so quickly in their later years. It feels like the inauguration was three months ago rather than three days ago. Or maybe it's the rapid proliferation of 10,000 Bernie Sanders mittens memes.

With a new administration in place, things are beginning to change for the better in terms of the federal response to the coronavirus pandemic. The administration has released its plan for bringing the plague under control.

The plan is a common-sense compendium of tried and true public health measures, most of which should have been in place last spring. It has taken the availability of vaccines into account, and there are now federal plans to utilize the National Guard and other elements of the government to get them out as quickly as they can be manufactured.

Locally, we here in Alabama are stymied by shortages in vaccine supply. The Alabama Department of Public Health, which controls all distribution in the state, has gotten its act together and is getting vaccines out to various points to begin vaccinating those over age 75. However, the complete lack of federal coordination has kept vaccines from flowing into the state to meet demand.

Vaccinators often don't know when they are going to get a shipment until a few hours before it arrives which makes setting up schedules and notifying patients a wee bit difficult. There are plans for several mass vaccination sites in the greater Birmingham area. The logistics are in place, but they can't open them up until there is a supply that can be counted on for both first and second shots.

><•••>

Numbers continue to mushroom.

There is some evidence that we have peaked and may be on the downward side of the hump caused by holiday gatherings and travel from Halloween through New Years. Numbers in the hospital locally are down slightly.

The percentage of positive tests is decreasing somewhat, but it is still more than double the 5% positive testing rule which is thought to be the level at which we can consider the pandemic under control in a particular area.

Anthony Fauci has finally been allowed to share his expertise with the public untrammeled. He is now responsive only to science and not to politics. His expression of delight—at being able to at long last speak unvarnished truth and swing the CDC and other health organizations toward protecting the public rather than protecting the optics of the White House—has been refreshing.

The next big issue is the spreading of the UK alpha variant which is significantly more contagious than the original strains. If this isn't slowed, we may barely get a rest from this peak before a whole other surge begins later this spring.

><•••>

Tonight was the one-year anniversary of the opening of the Virginia Samford Theater's production of *Cabaret*, the last live stage show I was part of during the "before" times. The cast gathered on Zoom to toast each other and watch an archival video of a performance.

I don't like watching myself in such things. Stage performances depend so much on the interaction of the actors with the audience that I always feel removed on both sides of the equation when it's on screen. However, it was fun to see everyone and to reminisce and comment on how appropriate that piece was to the political times we have been living in recently. When the local theater world opens back up, we're going to lobby for the theater to revive that production.

I've just started rehearsal on another project, a Zoom theater version of *Tartuffe* in which I'm playing Orgon. Now there's another play in sync with the times despite being 400 years old. That's what makes great art, something born of turbulent times that helps a future generation understand the chaotic swirl in which it finds itself.

>⊱

Bad times, pandemic disease, political unrest, religious schism—no society is immune from such things. We like to think of ourselves as privileged individuals living in the finest civilization the world has produced, an apogee of comfort and enlightenment. I'm pretty sure the Ancient Sumerians, the Imperial Romans, the Tudor British, the 18th century French, and all the others felt the same way about themselves and their societies in their day. I think it's part of the human condition to believe it can't happen here—until it does.

I have no idea how the new administration is going to go about solving the myriad problems in American society that our failed response to the coronavirus has exposed. I don't know what the opposition forces to President Biden and the Democratic party have planned in terms of response. All I can say is that there's going to be no linking arms around the campfire and singing *Kumbayah*.

We're a long way from controlling this pandemic. We must continue to be vigilant, vaccinated or not. Hundreds of thousands have died, hundreds of thousands more are likely to die, but we can all take simple steps to protect each other.

You know what to do. Stay home, wash your hands, wear your masks, and socially distance.

WEDNESDAY | JANUARY 27, 2021

I T'S WEDNESDAY AGAIN.

Three weeks ago on Wednesday, the Capitol was attacked. Two weeks ago on Wednesday, the previous president was impeached for a second time. One week ago on Wednesday, the new president was inaugurated. I'm kind of disappointed something momentous didn't occur today as well.

There's still a couple of hours left before midnight, unless you're east of Nova Scotia, so I suppose it's possible we'll have something major before the end of the day, but it may be that it's just as well that the Rule of Three is holding and we're all being given a chance to catch our collective breath.

We've all had a lot to absorb and process these last few months and I, for one, could use a little downtime. I don't know how the generation that made it through World War II was able to keep it up for six years.

The news is mixed from Covidland.

COVID hasn't gone away despite having been driven off the front pages recently by political news. It looks like the surge fueled by the holidays is starting to recede. Numbers are down in general.

Here at UAB, inpatients are down about 25% from a peak of near 300 to about 220. It's still far too many, and the numbers, in general, remain grim.

Worldwide, the count has broken nine figures with over 100 million cases recorded, likely an undercount by a significant margin.

>⊷≡

In the US, we're at about 25.5 million.

The speed with which we're experiencing new cases and deaths has begun to slow. Whether that's due to behavior change, vaccine distribution, or other reasons is not yet clear.

On the bad side, the new UK alpha variant that's significantly more contagious is definitely spreading in the US, and this may be enough to knock numbers back the wrong way again. Even here in Alabama, several cases of the new strain have been identified.

Vaccines are finally being more appropriately distributed. Every day I hear from a friend or a patient that they've received their first dose and are scheduled for their second. Systems are falling into place at both the federal and state levels to keep supplies up, the current limiting factor.

My VA house call program has solved the logistical problems related to transporting vaccine during its safe post-thaw window to our bed-bound house call patients around the state, and we are getting them slowly but steadily taken care of. (Large sigh of relief.)

There's still a lot of work to be done to reach and educate underserved communities, and there's still significant political stigma associated, but that seems to be waning somewhat as vaccines roll out with minimal side effects.

>⊷≡

It has been gratifying for me to see the return of the house call to a more prominent place in medical practice in recent years. I have always believed that they are central to helping people maintain good health.

Back in the day, before my time, most primary care medicine was done in the home. The doctor made the rounds in a mule cart or a

Model T. He, or more infrequently she, treated what he could be treated, educated families in proper nursing, and provided comfort when there wasn't much else available.

Following World War II, doctors migrated into offices, usually attached to hospitals in some way, so they could care for both outpatients and inpatients at the same time. They still did occasional house calls. The introduction of the federal payment structures of Medicare and Medicaid and the rise of for-profit insurance nearly killed them completely with a growing emphasis on time, efficiency, and volume.

When I entered medicine in the 1980s, there were no opportunities to observe or learn about the art of the house call. I was never exposed to one, even with my wandering around rural communities as part of the University of Washington's program to create primary care doctors with roots in small-town Northwest America.

Neither house calls nor geriatrics were part of my curriculum either in medical school or in residency. I didn't meet a geriatrician until I was nearly finished with my internal medicine training.

When I opted for geriatrics, one of my first assignments was to UC Davis's small outpatient geriatrics clinic. On one of my first weeks there, the ambulance pulled up and offloaded a poor lady on a stretcher. She couldn't get out of bed at home.

The process of transferring her from the bed to the ambulance and then into the clinic had aggravated her arthritis and she was crying from pain. She was demented and not able to tell me much of anything about her condition. No member of her family had come with her. The ambulance drivers knew little about her other than the address from which they had picked her up.

I called her home and reached her daughter. She hadn't been allowed in the ambulance and didn't have access to a car to come on her own. Through her I learned a bit about the patient. When I asked where the family lived, I discovered that it wasn't more than a few miles from my house. I told them that next time the patient needed medical care, I was going to come to them.

I had no idea how to do a house call. I went to the powers that be at UC Davis and told them I intended to do them on certain clinic patients who would otherwise require ambulance transport. There was no objection.

I located a group, the American Academy of Home Care Physicians, and attended their annual meeting looking for ideas. It fit in a classroom as there were fewer than 50 members nationwide.

I learned that the reason there were so few house calls was due to the Medicare reimbursement scale for physicians which, at that time, made it financially unfeasible to do them. As a fellow in an educational program, this wasn't an issue. I learned by doing. I did more.

I started to realize how much I missed out on by only seeing patients in the artificial environment of the clinic setting. And how much else there was to learn.

I discovered the family where all the medications were poured into a candy dish and grandma picked out the ones she felt like that day. I learned to equate chronic GI issues with unsanitary kitchens and help teach patients food safety. I learned to carry a large bottle of Febreze and spray myself down after visiting certain homes so I wouldn't smell like an ashtray the rest of the day. I learned how not to touch the furniture in some places. I put up with the occasional case of scabies from unwashed bed linens.

By the time I left Sacramento, I had built a thriving academic house call practice that taught house call medicine to residents and medical students and provided care to a uniquely vulnerable population. I became comfortable with people on ventilators at home and with families that more or less ran an ICU out of their kitchen.

Unfortunately, the program disappeared in the collapse of clinical geriatrics at UC Davis which forced me to leave California in search of alternate employment, but when I got to Birmingham, I brought that skillset with me.

The Birmingham VA had a functional home care service that I became part of for a while. I'm back with it again after a decade-long hiatus for other projects.

I introduced the UAB system to house calls and more or less did them on my own hook for years and years as they were the right thing to do. UAB eventually saw the wisdom in them and has built a robust house call service over the last few years. For the most part, however, I haven't been involved. I've simply had too much on my plate.

Going into someone's home as a physician gives me a unique perspective on a patient. I start to learn about who they are as people and what's important to them. I meet their families. I meet their pets. I meet their ancestors and learn their family histories from the pictures on their walls.

Most importantly, I meet them on their own turf. The power relationship is reversed. They are the ones in charge of what will and will not happen. There are times when I wouldn't have it any other way.

Sign up for your vaccine when you can. Even if you've gotten it, you know what to do: wash your hands, wear your mask, social distance, and don't take random pills out of a candy dish.

SUNDAY | JANUARY 31, 2021

I'S THE LAST DAY OF JANUARY, the end of the first month of this new year. And what a month it has been politically.

I would like to think that things will start to settle down into the old patterns where the news out of DC simply drones on in the background of life, but I'm not so sanguine as all that these days.

We've got an impeachment trial, an ex-president who has spent all his time in politics shattering norms and is almost certainly going to continue to do so, and a major political party unable to police itself against spokespeople minimizing sedition, nattering on about "Jewish space lasers," and doing nothing to dispel the Big Lie that the recent election was stolen. Forces that have been rending the social fabric won't be going away any time soon.

I'm no expert in politics, but I've studied my history and had a career that's brought me into contact with people from all walks of life. It's one that's required me to develop my sense of empathy far beyond where it once was and, once you have it, you can't really turn it off.

Emotions, especially negative ones like anger, are still running high. There's a strong belief that our government no longer works to support ordinary citizens.

On the left, this takes the form of government as a rigged game benefiting the wealthy at the expense of others which is playing out in the Game Stop short-sell market where some have figured out how to leverage technology to beat Wall Street.

On the right, it takes the form of government taking hard-earned tax dollars and giving them to the lazy "other" which is playing out in nativist and white nationalist sentiments.

It doesn't matter which side you're on. If enough of the population loses faith in the government for any reason, the government will eventually collapse, and we will be left to forge something different.

Periods of revolution and reformation are often violent. I have no interest in living through one, so let's all put our faith in understanding that government, of any stripe, is the mechanism by which we help each other beyond the circle of our immediate acquaintance.

Big problems like pandemics require big solutions that can only be provided through government. No other human institution is large enough.

The long and short of it is that we're in interesting times, as the old curse goes, and they're going to stay interesting for a while.

On the public health front, things are a bit easier locally. The number of hospitalized COVID cases continues to descend, albeit slowly. The rate of increase is not what it was a month ago, but it's still a good deal higher than it should be.

Vaccines are rolling out, and vaccination centers will start taking everyone over 65 as of February 8th. A number of high-risk occupations are also becoming eligible such as teaching and working in food service and retail.

Our local metro area has a number of mass sites up and running, the only limiting factor being supply of vaccine. There are still some issues to be worked out such as the classism of relying on sign-up systems that require online registration.

I like writing stories, but I've never been good at writing sustained narrative fiction. Like all of us, I feel like I have the great American novel inside me somewhere, but I've never been able to get out more than a chapter or two before running out of gas or being sidetracked by some other project.

Short-form has always worked better for me: these *Accidental*

Plague Diaries, for example, and the insane world of Mrs. Norman Maine and her movie reviews (which can currently be found at movierewind.com).

The one place I have been able to write long-form fiction has been in playwriting. I have a number of plays under my belt, some of which have gone on to independent life.

I started playwriting back in the 1980s when I was in medical school. An old friend from Stanford had also ended up in Seattle after completing both undergraduate and Stanford Law. We had collaborated before in college, most notably when she directed and I assistant directed *Hello, Dolly!* for the spring mainstage musical her senior year.

In the late 80s, she had this idea for an educational musical that could teach legal concepts to high schoolers. She got some grant funding, we sat down to write the book and lyrics together, found a composer, and *Whadda 'Bout My Legal Rights?* was born. It had grant money attached, so The Empty Space Theater picked it up for an Equity tour through Washington high schools (it was about 50 minutes long, designed to fit in an assembly period), and it's still available from Samuel French should any of you wish to produce it.

Our next collaboration was a farce, *Terrorist in the Family Room,* which we drafted out together character and plot-wise. But then I returned to California for residency while she stayed in Seattle, so she moved on to other projects. I rewrote and finished *Terrorist* and send it out occasionally to see if anyone wants to do it.

While everyone loves the script, it's never been produced. I should get it out again and do another rewrite for the age of Trump. The central idea that the terror we wreak on ourselves is far worse than what terrorists can do to us is resonating again. People think that the title refers to the main character, an international terrorist taken in by a suburban family by mistake. It actually refers to the TV set. Perhaps I need to change that to social media.

Ten years or so ago, I was asked to write some scripts for touring productions for the local senior theater group, *The Seasoned Performers*. These plays were specifically designed for elder actors to perform for elder audiences, predominantly in senior living facilities and senior centers. Being the good geriatrician that I am, I dutifully went to look up what there was on writing for senior audiences but didn't find much. So I turned to what I knew from decades of working with older generations, including how to communicate with those with hearing or visual impairments, how to work with those with mild cognitive issues, and generational concerns.

The result was two scripts. The first was *Grimm and Bear It*, a fantasy in which the traditional fairy tale villains, including the wicked witch, the big bad wolf, the troll, and the evil stepmother, are tossed out of their stories and made to wait together in the green room of the eternal theater while cultural forces beyond their control try to reshape the power of narrative. They escape with the help of the audience by breaking the fourth wall.

The second, *Nightcall Nurses,* had older actresses from a radio drama of that name coming back to the studio as honored guests, recognizing that they're being belittled for being older, and taking over the broadcast on their terms. I always thought I should write one more and then publish them as three plays for senior theater.

In between, I've written more editions of *Politically Incorrect Cabaret* than I can shake a stick at. I've wanted to write something serious for the stage, but I always seem to veer off into snide humor.

When I write comedy, I write it for me and for jokes I find funny, even if no one else gets them. For instance, in the very first *Politically Incorrect Cabaret*, we did a spoof of *The Trojan Women* as if they were survivors of the Iraq war. It was the middle of the Bush years, so Andromache had the following line: "We're getting our own *No Child Left Behind* program. They're starting with my son, Astyanax." I thought it was hysterical, but it probably went right over the heads of 99% of the audience.

These *Accidental Plague Diaries,* too, are written for me, to help me understand a changing and changed world through the power of narrative. I'm happy so many of you have jumped on for the ride. In the meantime, wash your hands, wear your masks, keep your distance, and tell the story.

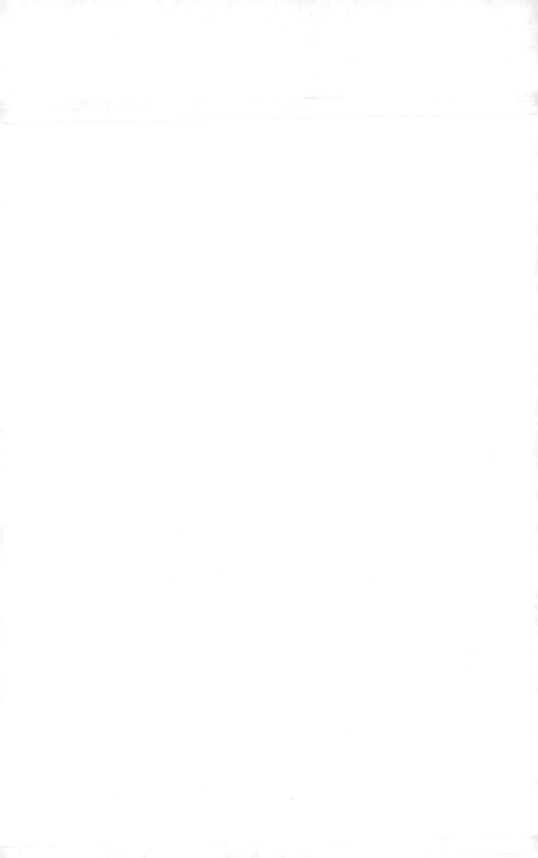

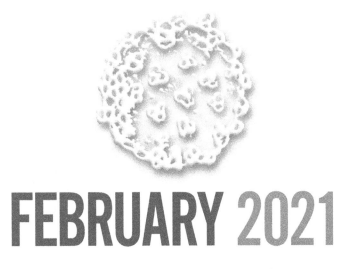

FEBRUARY 2021

Down in the Depths

WEDNESDAY | FEBRUARY 3, 2021

THE HOLIDAY SURGE IS OFFICIALLY OVER.

Case rates have dropped back to where they were in mid-November when the rise began to take off, a couple of weeks after Halloween parties. Back then, we were at roughly 10 million total cases and 240,000 US deaths. Now we're at 26.5 million cases and 450,000 US deaths.

More than 15 million people sick and more than 200,000 dead because America wasn't willing to stay home for the holidays.

I'm being a bit unfair. If we had all stayed home, there would still have been some cases, maybe a quarter or a third of those totals. We're still looking at a lot of people who didn't have to die but did because of our social hubris and lack of empathy.

Is the drop-off due to human behavior or due to the vaccine finally starting to roll out in significant quantities? Probably a bit of both.

About 5% of the eligible US population has been vaccinated. The emphasis on the high-risk populations of healthcare workers and elders in congregate living will significantly affect mortality rates.

While the numbers are still difficult to comprehend (roughly 1/730 Americans who were alive a year ago have died of COVID at this point), I'm starting to feel hopeful that we're going to have a bit more normal life come summer.

The local vaccination sites are working well. The only limiting factor is the supply of vaccine. My sources within the federal government tell me that there's a huge effort within the new administration to get those bottlenecks ironed out as soon as possible.

Many of my clinic patients are in the pipeline to get their shots, and we are getting shots hand-delivered to my house call patients. I may be able to get back on the road to see them over something other than a computer screen in a couple of months.

When I began these *Accidental Plague Diaries* in March of 2020, I had no intention of them being anything other than what they were: my musings on life, the universe, and everything, and a way of trying to make sense of my place in it. But when the whole of society was upended and everyone was as uncertain as I, it became clear that I had a gift for putting those existential fears into words, finding the threads of hope, and explaining the concepts we all needed to know in order to understand both the disease and the societal responses.

The feedback I received kept me writing until it dawned on me that I was accidentally writing a plague diary. Eventually, I realized I was writing a book about the coronavirus, both the government and the health system's responses, and what that meant to one man both inside and outside of health care.

If you'd told me back then that I would publish a first volume of these musings last August, and today be looking forward to publishing a second, I would have thought you were smoking something.

I'm taking time out for another Zoom theater piece, Moliere's *Tartuffe*. I first read it in high school and was amazed at how sharp the satire of religious hypocrisy was in something written centuries ago. It was one of those things that helped me understand that while culture and the trappings of society may change, humans remain fundamentally the same. I get the same feeling from Shakespeare and Sophocles. *Plus ça change, plus c'est la même chose.*

I've only seen *Tartuffe* staged once, at a small theater in Berkeley when I was a college student. When I picked it up to study it for this filming (I'm playing Orgon, the wealthy fool who takes in Tartuffe and is fleeced by him), I was struck by how relevant it is to our time.

A certain segment of religious America has hitched its wagon to irreligious charlatans for the promise of wealth and political power and, as the church is pulled away from its principles for temporal ends, the hypocrisy gap widens, diminishing both church and state. I think we're learning the lesson that in a pluralistic society, both church and state are stronger when they leave each other alone.

>——

I did some acting in elementary school. My first major role was as the title character in *Rumpelstiltskin* as I was the smallest boy in the third grade capable of memorizing the lines. I was a tiny child and the Saunders genome is wired in such a way that the males don't grow until relatively late. I was the smallest boy in my grade level all through elementary and middle school, remaining under five feet until I finished 8th grade (I shot up that summer).

Being very small in middle school and having a reasonable intellect was socially problematic, so I convinced myself that one of my best defense strategies was to be invisible and not make waves. (It didn't keep me from being thrown in the dumpster; I was just so easy to pick up.) Being invisible meant staying off stage. I entered high school not interested in performing but still enamored of the process of theater, so I became a techie and moved from that to stage management and eventually to directing.

Sometimes I wonder what my life might have been like if I had been a different person and had started performing at a younger age. Would I still have gone to med school or would I have tried the NYC thing to see if I had what it takes? Who am I kidding? I would still have gone to med school.

As much as I love the theater, I made the decision around age 20 that I always wanted to have it as an avocation and a love, and never feel like it was work. I also didn't want to tie my life to a profession that's more about being the right person in the right place at the right

45

time than it is about actual ability. Of course, there has been a certain amount of the former in my medical career anyway. Sometimes it has worked in my favor. Sometimes it hasn't.

I'm looking forward to getting back on stage. It's not ego-driven. Tommy always accused me of seeking the spotlight but I really don't care if I have a lead or am third nobody from the left. I enjoy the process of creation with a team of people, each bringing their individual skills, both on stage and off, to create something ephemeral that none of us could have possibly done on our own.

I choose the projects I get involved with based on the other people involved. There are people I like spending time with, people I want to learn from, people whose talent I admire. If there's a critical mass of that going on, sign me up and stick me where you need me.

I'm hoping there will be some outdoor distanced theater this summer and that we may be at a point where we can all gather again indoors in the fall. There are way too many shows on my bucket list that I want to be a part of before I become too infirm to run around backstage platforms in the dark changing clothes as I go.

Get Andy back on stage again! You know what to do to make it happen. Wash your hands. Wear your mask. Social distance. Stay out of crowds. Get your vaccine when you can.

SATURDAY | FEBRUARY 6, 2021

ONE YEAR. 366 DAYS (2020 WAS A LEAP YEAR). 527,040 minutes (Sorry, Jonathan Larson, but you're wrong every fourth year). It was initially assumed that the first US COVID death happened on February 29, 2020 in the Puget Sound area. But, when the pandemic began to take off in March, the medical examiner's office went back to a couple of mysterious unexplained deaths in otherwise healthy people following a flu-like illness and found the presence of the novel coronavirus in tissue samples of individuals who died on February 6th and February 17th. One year later, according to the Johns Hopkins Coronavirus counter, the US is at 460,311 deaths.

How big is that number? If it was a US city, it would be 44th in population, coming between Virginia Beach and Long Beach, CA. It's 10% higher than US World War II casualties, making the pandemic the third largest mass casualty event in US history, bested only by the Civil War and the 1918 Flu pandemic. It's enough to fill the 101,821 seats at Bryant Denny stadium four and a half times. It's enough to have killed one out of every 719 Americans who were alive a year ago.

As the average American has a circle of acquaintance of roughly 5,000 individuals, statistically each of us has lost seven people who were in our lives a year ago. For me, it's a much larger number than that given the nature of my profession. I lost seven people of my acquaintance during the first week of January alone as the surge driven by holiday gatherings reached its peak.

❧

Fortunately, things are beginning to calm down somewhat.

Numbers of hospitalizations, at least locally, are beginning to dwindle. There is one outlier, Tuscaloosa. I was in a meeting at the

VA this past week where there was much consternation about a rapid spike of COVID among veterans at the Tuscaloosa VA compared to the rest of the state. All you have to do to explain it is look to the night of January 11th when the Crimson Tide clinched the national football title and the young people of Tuscaloosa poured into the streets to celebrate.

⊷⊚

Human behavior drives the patterns of viral outbreaks in predictable ways. Most of those young people did not become seriously ill, and most elderly veterans in the area were not chugging beers on University Boulevard in the wee hours of the morning.

The mass of assembled people, however, allowed for the virus to be passed along to a greater portion of the population at one time. With higher numbers infected and a greater reservoir of potential carriers, older people in the community were more likely to come into contact with someone infectious, even with normal precautions.

With vaccine rolling out in fits and starts, there's a sense of societal ennui regarding COVID. I can't quite put my finger on it, but it's sort of an "OK, that's over, let's move on" sensibility which fits in neatly with both our short attention spans and need for the new, especially within the infotainment journalism we've perfected over the last few decades. COVID is so 2020. Let's move on to the next big story.

The problem is that the virus hasn't gone anywhere. It's just waiting for us to change our behaviors in ways it can exploit to do its one and only job: propagate. When we allow it to move through the population, we create two major issues. The first is the obvious cost of morbidity and mortality. The second is that we give the virus a chance to encounter more types of humans and more environments, thus increasing the chance of mutations.

Viruses are relatively simple organisms. There aren't a lot of pieces, so the genetic code isn't all that long. Errors in the transcription of genetic code happen all the time—anything from 1/100 to 1/1,000,000,000 depending on the organism and whether it's DNA, RNA, or mRNA.

The more different environments the virus encounters, the more likely one of those mistakes is going to turn out to be an evolutionary win in a new situation and give a new strain a little bit of an advantage. A win for the virus may well be a loss for us.

The novel coronavirus that causes COVID is very closely related to the virus that caused SARS in Asia a couple of decades ago. If a mutation occurs that causes this one to develop the same lethality as SARS, we may be in a world of hurt. SARS' mortality rate was about 14% compared to about 2% for COVID. With that level of morbidity, we'd be looking at between 3.5 and 4 million dead in this country to date.

I'm not pooh-poohing the vaccine at all. It's an incredibly useful tool and a tribute to human ingenuity that it got from identification of the virus into people's arms in less than a year. But it's not the be-all and the end-all, and it cannot substitute for good public health practices. It's going to take a while to get everyone at higher risk from COVID vaccinated—it's somewhere between 1/3 and 1/2 of the population.

The other things we've been working on such as masking, hand hygiene, and social distancing need to continue for a little while longer. It's still a bit unclear as to what is safe and what is not once you've received your vaccine. I'm still not eating out or going to the movies, but I feel better getting together with a couple of people, especially if we've all been vaccinated. I need a weekend away for mental health in the near future, somewhere where I can do outdoorsy things.

───⊶

We've still got a huge problem in this country when it comes to public health. The change in administration, while it did put people who will listen to and follow the science in charge of the pandemic response, did nothing to change the gap between red and blue America.

I think the most dangerous thing that can happen over the next year is for the administration and blue America to dismiss the concerns and attitudes of the anti-maskers and their ilk as insignificant noise coming from a bunch of uneducated yokels. The analysis of the composition of the mob at the Capitol shows that these are not uneducated or unsophisticated people.

This morning I read an article that the governor of Iowa is eliminating all social distancing, masking, and other coronavirus mitigation measures. One does not get to be a governor of any state by being a stupid person. But one does make political calculations based on various competing agendas.

I'm afraid our political split is here to stay unless some significant social surgery is performed (reinstatement of the fairness doctrine, repeal of Citizens United). I am under no illusions that things are over, not by a long shot

The Republican Party is in thrall to a radicalized base where any attempt at comity is seen as heresy. As that base pulls itself further and further into a world of "alternative facts," I have no idea what the leadership is going to do or what the economic powers behind the leadership are going to do.

My guess is, as radicalization becomes bad for business, politicians attempting to use those impulses for their advantage will start to see funding sources dry up until they fall back into line. But you never know.

It always comes down to money in our culture; it's the only common language. The later millennials and Gen Z folks seem to have figured this out—witness a group of Florida high schoolers eviscerating the National Rifle Association and a bunch of tech bros using the Robin Hood App to bring a hedge fund to its knees.

I feel like I'm blathering on a bit now so I'll sign off, but not without my usual litany. Wash yo hands. Wear yo mask. Stay yo distance. Get yo vaccine.

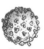

TUESDAY | FEBRUARY 9, 2021

WASN'T GOING TO WRITE AN ENTRY TONIGHT but when I opened up my laptop after work, some siren song seduced me into starting into the woods again.

I've been doing this long enough now to know that when the muse calls, you better answer because those half-formed ideas at the back of your brain won't be there when you look for them later. I've always written best by just letting my brain go into a sort of detached zone where I'm not really thinking, just letting the words come as they will.

When I write these essays, I sometimes have an idea or two. Sometimes a whole paragraph is in mind. Other times, I just start writing, and off we go. It's a bit of a dissociative state that lasts usually about 75 minutes or so, and then I find that there are 1200-1500 words on the screen. I don't rewrite. I hit post and hope for the best.

It's been interesting going back as I edit these *Accidental Plague Diaries* into book form. They weren't written with that in mind and the chore of analyzing the ideas in each one, making sure there's a certain stylistic and thematic unity, getting rid of odd tangents, the occasional major grammatical error, misspelling, or unfortunate word choice is teaching me a lot about what my writing actually is.

My editor asked me the ultimate question in our last conference. Why is such a book important?

I want it to be a primary source document of a particular moment in history written as that history was unfolding from the perspective of someone with some understanding of both the health and sociological implications that are happening all around, and the impact the coronavirus had on both one person and on the country as a whole.

We'll see if I manage to actually do that.

There's not a lot to report from the battlefield over the last few days. The number of hospitalized cases continues to dwindle locally as the holiday-fueled surge continues to recede. UAB Hospital, which topped out at about 300 inpatients at the peak, is down to just over half that at the moment.

I am breathing a major sigh of relief as this means it is unlikely I will be called into work for inpatient duty later this month. If I *was* called in, my plan was to go in, tell the residents that I hadn't really done this sort of work since before they were born (not quite true), and to please lead me gently by the hand through anything for which they needed staff authorization.

The vaccination centers are also apparently working relatively well. I see more and more friends outside of health care proudly holding up their vaccination cards on social media. We just need to get more vaccine into the state faster. We've also got to keep working against some of the more ridiculous disinformation circulating out there.

Tyler Perry did a very good PSA on the vaccine aimed at the African-American community (it's on YouTube) which does a nice job dispelling many of the worst myths. The most worrying thing at the moment is the rapid spread of the UK alpha strain that is much more infectious. It's currently doubling in prevalence roughly every ten days. At that rate, it will be 1,000 times as prevalent in three months and nearly 10,000 times as prevalent in four. (Ah, the magic of exponents.)

⚬

The creators of modern myths were on full display today as the curtain rose on *Impeachment 2: Electric Boogaloo.*

It's quite something when the second-worst performance by an attorney on a given day involved a Zoom court appearance and a cat filter. I try to be evenhanded in my approach to politics, but I'm having grave difficulties listening to even sound bites from the pundits trying to gaslight me into believing that the Capitol Insurrection was not what it was.

The ceremonies will play out. There will be some sort of legalistic coda. But nothing will really change as nothing has been done about the media and political landscape that has let untruths and half-truths flourish to the point of having two societies trying to coexist with alternative facts. I don't know how to fix it. All I can do is try and understand it.

⚬

I was thinking about our divided society and how to really grasp what it means when I realized it's something I deal with every day, only in microcosm. Perhaps the most common serious health problem for which I am consulted is cognitive change. The memory loss that afflicts the aging is usually, but not always, a dementing illness. It's relatively uncommon before the age of 75 and then starts to rise exponentially. The Baby Boom generation is just starting to enter the dementia years this year.

Prevalence of significant memory loss is less than 10% at age 75, 20% at age 80, 40% at age 85, 60% at age 90, 80% at age 95, and pretty universal at age 100. There is plenty of evidence that if all humans lived long enough, we would all develop Alzheimer's type dementia. There's even some evidence that it's a lifelong process, wired into our central nervous system's design—the price we pay for our intellects.

In previous generations, the majority died of other causes long before it would have become apparent. Will the Boom, still considering themselves young in their late 60s and early 70s, and living to age in reasonable health, be able to cope with the combination of physical health and cognitive failure?

An interesting thing happens to long-term married couples where one partner develops dementia with age and the other does not. The well partner is usually the last to come to grips with the changes and deficits in their spouse. Alzheimer's type dementia is usually of such slow onset and progression that the well spouse unconsciously adapts to that change, taking on more and more life tasks without necessarily understanding that they are doing so.

It's the child who lives out of state, who hasn't been home in several years and arrives for the holidays, who can truly see the changes because of the delta between what they expect to see and what they do see.

Once the spouse starts to understand that their partner is not reacting to them in the way they are used to, they try all the techniques a lifetime of marriage has taught them in terms of cajoling, fighting, teaching, and just being. These techniques tend to fail. So they double down, try even harder, and get the opposite results of what they expect. Eventually, they show up in my office angry, frustrated, resentful, sad, and not understanding why the dynamics of their relationship aren't working the way they think they should.

It's my job to begin the process of teaching them that the demented spouse lives in a different reality with different rules. Time may not exist in the same way. They may both look at the same thing but see something different as the demented brain may interpret signals in unusual patterns.

Reality is what our brains tell us it is. As most of our brains function in roughly the same way, we agree on it or, as Lily Tomlin once put it,

"Reality is a collective hunch." When a brain no longer functions in the same way, reality becomes different. That person no longer lives in our world. We aren't really capable of visiting their world either.

There are tantalizing clues as to what the world of dementia is like. When we look at the work of demented visual artists, for example, we see that they pick strong and vibrant colors and simplify line and detail. Other people strip away adult dissimulation and artifice and become plainspoken and absolute truth-tellers.

It's no accident that in classical literature the fool is always the one who speaks truth to power. Shakespeare brings it all together in *King Lear* when the king and the fool confront the storm on the heath. Lear is a portrait of dementia robbing a powerful man of independence, but not self-awareness, and the fool is the one person who understands him. The relationship between Lear and his daughters plays out in my waiting room about once a week as adult children try to figure out what to do with daddy as he's losing his faculties.

><⊚

Our current society is like a long-term couple where one partner has dementia. I won't say which one. People of different political persuasions will pick different sides, but the analogy holds either way.

Red America and blue America are trying to exist in two different realities. The relationship is frustrated and foundering because they're trying to use the same old communication methods to get through to each other. All it's doing is raising the level of anger.

Perhaps we could use some advice from a friendly geriatrician, take a step back, not try to force each other into old roles, but gently explore who we are as new and evolving people in a spirit of mutual respect. Some of my usual suggestions, like distracting each other with cookies to help change brain patterns aren't going to work, but an acknowledgment that we have to move forward toward new ways of rapprochement might be useful.

We're going to have to do something to get us all on the same page regarding public health if we really want to bring COVID to task. In the meantime, wash your hands, wear your mask, keep your distance, get your shot, have a cookie.

SATURDAY | FEBRUARY 13, 2021

ANOTHER SATURDAY NIGHT AND I AIN'T GOT NOBODY. I think somebody else sang that first. And it's not entirely true this evening. Anastasia the cat is snuggled up to my feet on the bed as I write this, purring away while Oliver is yowling in the next room, hoping I'll get up and give him more kitty treats as if I didn't give him a few an hour ago.

Tommy's been gone nearly three years now and people are kindly sidling up to me asking when I'm going to date seriously again. I don't know. Next week? Next month? Next year? Next decade? I don't feel any particular compulsion to pair up again, except when it's Valentine's Day Eve and my social media is full of pictures of the happy couples of my acquaintance.

Dating in the gay world is hard. There's not a lot of social support for gay male romance, especially in my age group.

The last time I went through all this, 20 years ago, the number of eligible men local to Birmingham was rather small. Prior to meeting Tommy, I had been dating a man who lived in Michigan. We would meet for the weekend once a month or so somewhere in between.

Tommy fell into my life in an odd way. We had been chatting online, he had called me up in my professional capacity to gather information on elder care for a grant proposal he was writing for his job at Birmingham Health Care, and he started turning up at church where he was good friends with some other congregants.

When I figured out it was the same guy turning up in all these different areas of my life at the same time, I decided the universe was trying to tell me something, so I asked him out. The rest, as they say, is history. It did lead to a very public courtship with the entire congregation of the Unitarian Universalist Church of Birmingham egging us on. If the right guy turns up again in a similarly serendipitous manner, I'll consider a third husband, but I'm not going to actively look.

COVID is, of course, making dating nigh on impossible. There's no going out to dinner, or for drinks after work, or to the movies. I suppose a day hike together through one of the local mountain parks is a possibility, but it's a bit chilly for that. Maybe later in the spring.

In the meantime, I have all my various home projects plus a few extra work things I've taken on to supplement my salary that has this mysterious way of going down rather than up these days due to the crazy impact of the current crisis on the fiscal underpinnings of medicine.

I spent most of today wrestling with 2500 pages of medical records for a legal case in defense of a nursing home. Next week, I get to figure out how to collapse all I know about geriatric syndromes into a 75-minute lecture for a national board review course. I suppose somebody has to do it, and it might as well be me.

The news on COVID continues to improve.

The numbers continue to fall from their peak five weeks ago, but they're hardly going away. We're up to 27.5 million cases and will surpass 500,000 deaths by the end of the month.

Our local system for vaccine distribution appears to be working well. I have heard nothing but rave reviews from my patients and their families for the efficiency with which the mass vaccination sites are operating at UAB and in Hoover at Hoover Met Stadium.

The only limitation is the flow of vaccine into the state, but that appears to be happening in a much more predictable fashion than it was a month ago. Most of my over-75 patients who want a vaccine have either had their first dose or are scheduled within the next couple of weeks. Every vaccine delivered is one more person who will not end up in the ICU in a month or two. This will give our frazzled health system and its providers a bit of breathing space.

As I read through the information on the Pfizer and Moderna vaccines and how they are performing, it's safe to say that they are doing a very good job at preventing illness and complications. It's less clear if they are preventing transmission.

Some data is coming in suggesting that they do indeed do this as well, but we'll have to wait for the data scientists to capture and crunch the numbers before any definitive statements can be made. If this is indeed true, we should be able to reduce our need for masking and social distancing this summer.

I just want to get back to rehearsal. So much of my social life and my equipoise is tied up in creating art with others, in the rehearsal room and on stage, that I feel incomplete without it. I even miss tech rehearsals, the kind where cast and crew look at each other in hour four and ask why they do this to themselves when it would be less painful to go out in the alley and beat each other with pointed sticks.

The political world today progressed exactly as predicted with a pretty much party-line impeachment acquittal of the former president. For good or ill, I don't think that particular story is over in the least. The fault lines remain. The former president, if true to character, will not remain quietly off the political stage, but will continue to try and exert his will through his usual methods. What that will lead to, I haven't the vaguest.

At the moment, my part of the medical world is just happy that the CDC is authoring recommendations that make scientific sense, the FDA is offering well-sourced information about treatment alternatives, and the powers of the executive are working together to get vaccines out in a streamlined fashion. I'll take it.

⤚⊷

I haven't told a story for a while as COVID has me looking for metaphors and connections between the pandemic and other areas of life rather than just thinking back on my past. Here's one from my early house call days.

I went out to take a look at a demented gentleman who kept getting burns on his toes. He and his family didn't have much money and lived in a rental home that might best be described as a tar paper shack.

Like a lot of older homes, it was heated in winter by gas heaters that were attached to the gas line with a rubber hose so that you could place the heater in various parts of the house. The joists and the floorboards were rotted, and it was somewhat tricky to pick your way through the living room without putting your foot through to the crawl space.

It didn't take long to figure out that the reason he was burning his toes was that when he complained of cold feet, the family wheeled him up to the heater, and his diabetic neuropathy prevented him from noticing when they got him a little too close.

He was eating badly and we needed to get a weight on him. He couldn't stand on his own and they only had a bathroom scale, so I weighed myself, and then, he being a small and somewhat emaciated man, I picked him up and stood on the scale so we could get his weight by subtracting out mine.

He peed all down my front as I had him in a honeymoon carry. Meanwhile, his wife (schizophrenic and refusing to take her meds)

59

was frying something up in the kitchen for breakfast. She reached up, opened a cupboard, and an enormous winged roach flew out and settled itself on the cooking. Without missing a beat, she picked up a can of Raid, sprayed the roach (which flew off elsewhere), the food, and the open flame of the gas stove with it.

Fortunately, there was no explosion but she did turn around and ask me if I would like to stay for the meal. I politely declined, finished my visit, and hightailed it back to the car for a clean T-shirt and my bottle of Febreze. Geriatrics: the glamour specialty.

Stay well, stay warm, stay distant, wear your mask, wash your hands, use your sanitizer—but keep it off your breakfast sausage.

TUESDAY | FEBRUARY 16, 2021

S NOW DAY! Or at least some white-stuff-on-the-ground and some ice-on-the-roads day.

I woke up this morning to white flakes drifting dreamily down past my windows, told the VA that they could call me if they needed me, rolled over, and went back to sleep for another four hours. I haven't been that busy or that active recently so I assume it was some sort of destressing mechanism on the part of my brain.

The last few hours were full of wild dreams including a visit to Disney in which I could not figure out how to get inside the park, a cruise to an unpleasant destination with even worse people, and a sequence where I kept breaking into my pastor's house to find a nice quiet place to read and recuperate. She kept coming home and chasing me out again, politely but firmly setting her boundaries for family time.

It would have been nice if I could have spent the snow day in some mindless activity, but alas a phone call from an attorney stating he needed a report in writing tomorrow on the case I have been reviewing put paid to that idea. I had to dive back into 2500 pages of mainly unreadable electronic health records trying to extract nuggets of fact that would support my opinions. Fortunately, I found what I was looking for, wrote up five pages, got it to him by close of business Eastern time, and now have the evening to myself.

I really should charge more for rush jobs. Reviewing medical records is nowhere near as fun as it was when I first started decades ago. Back then I would get a banker's box shipped parcel post full of barely legible photocopies of physician handwriting to decipher. Now I get access to a Dropbox account full of perfectly legible electronic records spat out by some computer, most of which are useless garbage, unhelpful when trying to reconstruct what happened around a particular incident or illness.

There has been some speculation that at least some of the issues of response to COVID and COVID vaccination are tied up in the electronic health record that has become so pervasive. The groundwork for such records was laid in the late 1990s after the invention of the World Wide Web. Medicine, along with other industries, embraced the opportunity for information exchange that this allowed. Bad actors early on who were buying and selling health information led congress to pass the Health Insurance Portability and Accountability Act (HIPAA) in 1996 under the Clinton presidency.

This law explicitly protected the privacy of health information so that it could not be used in inappropriate ways. Unfortunately, it also tied a lot of information exchange to 1990s technology which is why health care, as an industry, still depends on the fax machine. It's considered HIPAA compliant while newer methods of information exchange are not addressed in the legislation and it has yet to be updated.

In the early 2000s, various private companies began to get into the electronic health record business, knowing it would be the wave of the future. Cerner and Epic are the biggest, but there are lots of smaller ones out there.

The VA actually offered its in-house EMR, known as CPRS, free of charge to the country so that there could be a national standard and all records could be easily traded between states and institutions without difficulty. However, the Republican president and congress of the time preferred to let private enterprise take precedence over the public commons.

The idea of standardized health records was abandoned in favor of dozens of incompatible systems incapable of talking to each other, leading to a dramatic increase in siloing of health systems along information lines.

Another complicating factor regarding electronic health records involves what they are asked to do. When clinicians sold control of the health system to industry and administrators in the late 70s and early 80s, there was a shift in the power dynamic. Where before, the needs of the physician were paramount, the needs of the industry, as exemplified by revenue generation, became the most important thing in terms of data management.

As administrators were in charge of purchasing health information systems, they looked for systems that could assist with capturing charges, identifying utilization trends, and assisting with quality metrics. The actual needs of an individual provider/patient encounter became subservient to these big data analytic requirements.

Administrative systems were modified to fulfill clinical requirements instead of vice versa. This was all put on steroids by the HI-TECH legislation signed by Obama in 2009 as part of the recovery from the Great Recession where the healthcare industry was offered financial incentives to adopt electronic health records, and pretty much everyone went digital over the next decade, each in their own way.

The end result is millions of data points that can be spit out at the touch of a button, but none of the logical thinking and cohesiveness that a physician's mind uses to take all of that and turn it into an understandable narrative. A set of vital signs or a set of lab values taken in isolation doesn't mean much. This information needs to be combined with clinical reasoning skills, an understanding of the prior medical history of the patient, the unique circumstances of life surrounding the patient, and occasional serendipity in order to be made to mean anything.

You learn to look at voluminous records and recognize that there are only a few sections, those where a clinician is entering data by free text or dictation, that can really let you know what you need to know and, when meeting a new record system, learning where those few areas can be found makes all the difference.

In the 1980s, when I began in medicine, pretty much everything was handwritten. That's why doctors' penmanship is so notorious. It comes from years and years of having to write so much so fast. In the 1990s, handwritten notes tended to be interspersed with dictations, especially of summary notes such as admitting histories and discharge summaries.

When I first came to UAB, there was no centralized medical record on the outpatient side. If I wanted to know what cardiology was doing with one of my patients, I had to go down to the cardiology clinic, pull the right chart, and take a peek. That started to change in the early 2000s when more centralized records became the norm, with dictated notes being accessible throughout the health system and electronic medication lists coming into being which could be updated and modified by any provider.

In the 2010s, the full electronic health record went into play. Notes pull information in from various places in the system but, as it is done automatically, there's no real understanding of relevance. Many notes become pages and pages of extraneous numbers and information with no clinical bearing on care.

Who knows what the 2020s will bring? I'm hoping for systems programmed more to respond to clinical needs than administrative ones where physicians and other clinicians are part of the teams that develop the programming so that it becomes more intuitive.

><>

Back to the COVID issues.

As these systems are now everywhere but are decentralized, when a national emergency such as the current pandemic hits, it's difficult, if not impossible, to get health systems to pull together as one because their data systems are incompatible. As a UAB physician, I have no way of knowing what happens to my patients at St. Vincent's or in the Baptist system unless the providers there are kind enough to send me records of the visit. (It happens sometimes.)

These records can be scanned into the UAB system, but they cannot be converted into a format where the data can be taken up and integrated with UAB data. Life becomes interesting when I have a patient who wants to get their primary care from me but still sees their cardiologist at St. Vincent's, their endocrinologist at Brookwood, and their neurologist at Grandview.

With these fault lines, I don't know how the administrative folk at the Alabama Department of Public Health, or at the upper echelons at UAB, are supposed to coordinate their efforts. Nor do I know how well they are doing at vaccinating five million Alabamians, half of whom fall into a risk group of some sort. It's a minor miracle that things are going as well as they are.

><>

Many people remain angry that they or their loved ones have not yet been able to get scheduled for a COVID shot. The limitation is the amount of vaccine coming into the state. Given that it's a commodity with far more demand than supply, people are turning their frustration on each other: Why is so and so able to get a shot when I have not? Why is this risk group deemed more important than that risk group?

The anger is misplaced. It shouldn't be leveled at vaccine recipients. (It's this sort of divide-and-conquer feeling that keeps problematic social structures in place.) The anger should be leveled where it belongs: directly at the previous administration which did little to make the vaccine available in a timely fashion. Had they used the powers of the federal government back in December when the vaccines were first approved, to accelerate manufacture and to coordinate distribution, it's likely that everyone at risk would be vaccinated by now. They didn't, meaning that a true ramp-up of vaccine delivery didn't start until after the change in administration a month later.

We'll get there. I am very optimistic that those at significant risk will all be vaccinated by Easter. That's 40 days from now. (I know this because today is Mardi Gras or, given the temperatures outside, Mardi Froid might be more apropos.) It's going to take more than fractured information systems and the ineffectiveness of administrations past to keep the American people down.

In the meantime, you know what to do: keep your hands washed, keep your distance, keep your mask on, keep out of indoor locations with lots of other people, keep on keeping on.

SUNDAY | FEBRUARY 21, 2021

EVERYBODY TALKS ABOUT THE WEATHER, but no one does anything about it.

I wish I could take credit for that particular *bon mot,* but it's been floating around for more than a century, attributed to various Edwardian era wits, most frequently Mark Twain. Sometimes I think I missed my century; that I was born to sit around a splendid drawing-room in evening wear with a snifter of brandy and a cigar, trading epigrams with celebrated names.

Then I think of the general standards of public health and hygiene at the time and feel thankful to have come of age in post-war America. Besides which, I'm not nearly as witty on my feet as I like to think I am. I do my best when scripted or in character in some way. When I'm just being me, my general introversion and insecurities take over.

$\rightsquigarrow$

The weather here has been cold but relatively pleasant following the snow and ice of last Tuesday (which was gone by Wednesday). Not so much in Texas, where the deep freeze continues to bedevil the population with power outages and a lack of potable water.

If I understand things correctly, plans were drawn up ten years ago following the last bad winter storm to hit the state, but nothing was done to implement the recommendations. The wholesale transfer of the commons to private corporations for purposes of enriching stockholders has its predictable consequences.

This has been cast in political terms as a battle between capitalism and socialism, but it's really more about a battle between private greed and public good. To my mind, there are certain sectors of the economy that should be kept public and not-for-profit because when they become private for-profit concerns, the law of unintended consequences, hurts us all. These include health care, education, corrections, the military, and utilities.

>—⊙

On the COVID front, I remain cautiously optimistic.

The numbers continue to decline nationwide. No one is certain why. Is it the presence of vaccinated individuals interrupting transmission chains? The surge caused by holiday behaviors being finally behind us? The numbers of infected individuals rising as a percentage of the population? Some new and as yet unidentified factor? Inquiring minds want to know.

We are at 498,500 deaths today, meaning we will pass the half-million mark tomorrow or the day after, less than a year since the pandemic established itself in North America.

It's hard to understand what sort of number that is. It's big enough that the US as a whole lost a year of life expectancy during the first six months of 2020, something that hasn't happened in generations.

People don't really understand what that life expectancy number is. It's been hovering in the high 70s for the last couple of decades, inching up a bit here and there. It doesn't mean, obviously, that everyone only lives to that age. It's the statistical mean age to which the cohort of babies born in that year will live. So the babies born in the first half of 2020 can expect a year shorter life than those born in 2019 due to the impact of COVID on society.

Life expectancy is driven down by disease processes that kill the young. It was only in the mid-40s a century ago, not because people died of old age at 50, but because so many babies and children died of what, with public health measures and antibiotics, became preventable diseases.

COVID is a preventable disease with proper public health measures, but politics got in the way. We can tell that mitigation measures

67

are working, even the imperfect ones we have in place, by looking at this year's flu statistics. The number of flu cases this year is less than 1% of what is seen in a typical year. Social distancing and masking prevent influenza from being transmitted as well as COVID.

Tartuffe concludes filming this next week and will be available in mid-March for your amusement. I've auditioned for a few other projects and am waiting to hear. I'm also starting outdoor, socially distanced, and masked rehearsals for a condensed production of *The Pirates of Penzance* later this next week. I have not yet been informed if I am a pirate, a policeman, one of Major General Stanley's daughters—or perhaps all three.

Last night, I was the MC for the church's annual fundraising evening —on Zoom rather than live this year—19 years after I first did it (my first Birmingham acting gig and the first appearance of what became the *Politically Incorrect Cabaret* Ansager). I paid homage to previous years by continuously changing my coats. There's only so much you can do in front of a webcam.

Work has been somewhat busy the last few weeks with various minor projects coming due, so between those and theater, I've been pretty nose-to-the-grindstone and will be into early March.

I wrote a compelling essay on why you can't find a geriatrician for your aging parent which I will post, but it's embargoed until after it goes live on the website I wrote it for. You will all just have to wait.

In the meantime, keep those hands washed, those masks on, and that space between you.

THURSDAY | FEBRUARY 25, 2021

'M NOT KEEN ON EMOTIONS.

I don't understand them very well. When I feel something swell up inside me, I have a difficult time determining if it's something positive or negative and what my reactions should be to it.

I tend to draw back from it, get quiet, try to analyze it, and figure out just what it should be rather than letting go and just feeling it. Perhaps this underlies my affinity for Sondheim. So much of his writing is for characters trying to move from the outside of intellect and analysis to the inside of emotional connection.

Time to put on *Anyone Can Whistle* for the umpteenth time. At least I have a new recording of that score to enjoy courtesy of Jay records. It's also likely why my only successful romantic relationships have both been with men who were creatures of instinct and emotions strong enough to batter down all of my carefully constructed walls. Keep that in mind before you try and fix me up with someone.

I just know that at the moment I am feeling a combination of positive and negative things. Today was the first live in-person rehearsal I have had in nearly a year. I was bouncing up and down in my chair at work all day with excitement.

It's been a rare week that I've gone without a rehearsal or a performance of some sort since launching myself into my late-life performing career back in 2003, and it's now just two weeks short of a year since I last sat in a seat with other people and we joined our voices together to make music.

I'm playing one of the policemen in a truncated, outdoor version of *The Pirates of Penzance,* produced by Opera Birmingham, and going up at Avondale Amphitheater in April. We're rehearsing masked and outdoors. We're maintaining social distancing in both rehearsal and staging.

When we began to sing the counterpoint of *When The Foeman Bares His Steel* and *Go Ye Heroes*, I wanted to cry. It's my favorite piece of music from the show, and to be enveloped in those 150-year-old melodies with a group of people just as grateful to be there as I was is as special a moment as I have had in a while.

We're rehearsing in a covered parking garage so the acoustics aren't bad. The cast is talented and full of old friends. I can't wait until we have the next one. So, if you're around 6th Avenue South in Avondale in the next month or so, and you hear operetta drifting by on the wind, you'll know what's going on.

This feeling, which I suppose is joy, is getting thoroughly mixed up with another one which I suppose is sorrow as I continue to work through the impact of COVID on my world.

We're at 508,000 deaths, according to the Johns Hopkins Coronavirus Counter, out of 28.4 million US cases. We're still a few days from the first anniversary of a death from an observed US infection (February 29, 2020—the few deaths earlier were traced back months later using blood and tissue samples).

We'll end up somewhere around 510,000-515,000 deaths at the one-year mark—enough to be the 37th largest city in the USA between the population of Atlanta and Sacramento. That's roughly ten times the number of flu deaths in the worst flu years and 25 times the number of flu deaths in light years. Flu is practically non-existent this year. Our good health habits are keeping the usual flu viruses from propagating.

I know the devastating impact that the death of important people has had on my life. Those of you who have not been widowed have no idea how much that process turns your life and your world upside down.

This year has created hundreds of thousands of new widows. New single-parent families. New orphans. A new crop of parents burying their children before them. And all having to be done while navigating a myriad of new social customs and rules, many of which keep us from being together.

There are really only two things that heal grief: time and the presence of others in our lives. The latter has been hard to find. What does grief deferred do to an individual? To a society? I think back on the generations that survived World War II or the Civil War and wonder what lessons they have to teach us about coping in healthy ways.

Steve died 20 years ago this year.

That's a long time, and I've had a whole other life in those years, but I can still feel his presence, hear his voice and his laughter as if he had just left the room.

His death, as it was a prolonged process of several years, caused me to make some life decisions that continue to have repercussions. When he became ill and I needed to spend more time and energy at home with him, I took myself off the fast track to academic success, leaving behind research interests and the very long hours that would have been necessary to position myself where I would be competitive for the department chair and dean's level jobs.

Could I have done both? Possibly, but likely at significant cost to my humanity, so I didn't want to try. Plus, I had the added burden of being openly gay at a time when few medical school faculty were. Those in my generation learned early and often that if you were open, you had to be twice as good to get half the credit.

Steve's death boomeranged me into a different career trajectory, maybe not as rewarding in terms of money or professional accolades, but certainly more fulfilling, and it allowed me the time and the energy to become a fully realized human being with my rediscovery of theater under the tutelage of Tommy.

I'm sure Tommy's death has also pushed my life in a new direction that's not yet fully clear. I've made certain decisions about what's important in my professional and personal lives that made me decide that downsizing and simplifying were things I needed to do. They also have made me decide that pulling up stakes and trying to vault up the ladder somewhere else (something I was looking at together with Tommy prior to his death) is not likely to happen.

Tommy's been gone nearly three years now. That wound is far fresher, and there are times I mourn. For some reason, last night, rather than doing something constructive (sorry people to whom I owe that Topics in Geriatrics lecture), I opened his Facebook and scrolled through the whole thing back to 2007.

Was I feeling sorrow? Was I feeling joy at what was? Was I feeling nostalgic? I can't say. I just know that I was feeling. And I think it was brought about by a combination of the joy of impending rehearsal and the sorrow of being surrounded by so much death and despair. The feeling of being alive. (There goes Sondheim again, and I didn't even intend it.)

Be like the singers of Opera Birmingham. Wear your mask. (Singing through it is… interesting.) Wash your hands. Sit six feet apart. Make the world a better place with music.

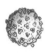

SUNDAY | FEBRUARY 28, 2021

AND THEN THERE WERE THREE.

We have a third vaccine available for COVID-19 approved for emergency use as of this weekend. It can be shipped and available for willing arms as early as tomorrow.

This one, from Johnson & Johnson, has several distinct advantages over previous vaccines from Moderna and Pfizer. It is a single-dose vaccine. Once you have your first shot, you're done. No need to return within the necessary window of time for a second. It's also much more stable and does not require the cold temperatures of the mRNA vaccines. It can be kept in an ordinary refrigerator.

This combination of factors will make it much easier to distribute, especially to more isolated populations. The homebound elders I take care of, outside of the VA which has a separate system, have for the most part been out of luck at obtaining vaccines. No good system for getting vaccines out to the community without compromising the cold chain had yet been devised locally. This will no longer be an issue.

The reason for this ease of use is that the Johnson & Johnson shot is a very different technology than that of the earlier vaccines. The two in circulation are based on a method of getting mRNA that encodes for spike proteins into our cells. This lets our own immune systems take over to produce antibodies against those proteins and, therefore, against the coronavirus.

The Johnson & Johnson vaccine works more akin to an inactivated virus vaccine such as for flu. This vaccine uses a modified adenovirus (a type of virus that causes a range of respiratory and GI viral illnesses) that cannot cause human illness. These viruses are DNA-based viruses (unlike the coronavirus which is RNA-based).

DNA that encodes for the spike protein is added to the adenovirus and, with the immunization, the introduced adenovirus is taken up by human cells. The virus itself is destroyed, but the DNA in question is taken up by the nucleus. The human cell makes mRNA for the spike protein which is recognized by the immune system as foreign. This primes the body to react against coronavirus should it be exposed later.

The numbers in regard to protection for the Johnson & Johnson vaccine aren't quite as spectacular as for the two prior vaccines but still plenty high enough to prevent significant illness in someone who is later exposed. Cold symptoms we can tolerate; shutting down of the respiratory system we can't.

With all three vaccines now approved and in circulation, we have a chance of getting ahead of the virus and its spread. We may be able to have a semblance of normal life again this summer. I'm dreaming of sitting on a patio with a cocktail and a bunch of friends having adult conversation.

The decline in cases nationally no longer continues to decline, but appears to have plateaued. The numbers are far below what they were at their January peak but they remain worse than they were in the early fall before cases really started to skyrocket.

I am not an epidemiologist but my guess is that the rapid fall was a result of picking the easy fruit. Rapid vaccination of seniors in congregate living is the likely driver as their chances of acquiring COVID and becoming seriously ill were so high. With that particular population stabilizing, we're probably looking now at numbers for the general population. Those will be much tougher to get under control, especially as roughly 1/3 of the adults in the country are living in a political fantasy land where such things as facts and how biology works don't matter.

The new variants which are more contagious continue to spread, but the vaccines appear to be as effective against them as they had been against original strains. Just to be on the safe side, the vaccine companies are working on boosters and tweaks should they be needed.

The biggest issue is one that has not yet reared its head but very well could. The coronavirus is a very simple organism genetically. Its RNA code consists of a small number of base pairs and very few parts. As RNA and DNA constantly mutate as nature tries things out (evolution exists whether you choose to believe in it or not), and those mutation rates are relatively constant, there will, over time, be more and more variants. Eventually one of those variants may develop a resistance to vaccine or a quality that makes it much more lethal to humans. If that starts to spread in the midst of our current political climate, there may be hell to pay.

><@

I haven't been feeling great the last couple of days. I'm pretty sure it's not COVID. UAB, however, from an abundance of caution, is going to test me in the morning and have me work from home tomorrow.

This is one of the few times since the pandemic broke that I haven't felt up to snuff. COVID avoidance has kept me away from all of the other mild ailments I usually get.

There is a code in medicine that you don't take sick time when you're under the weather as it means your workload will simply be added to someone else's when you're out. It's instilled during med school and residency which is full of stories about residents putting in their own IVs and making their rounds dragging an IV pole when they've been so sick and dehydrated they can barely stand up.

These stories are told in such a way as to make trainees feel that they should have a constitution of iron and that they are unworthy if they don't. I'm not sure that's a healthy attitude and I'm pretty sure I've gotten or given viral illness to and from colleagues and/or patients in the past. Maybe a gift of the current pandemic is a change in the culture to make it a positive move to stay home when we are sick and thus lessen the chances of iatrogenic infection.

Checklist for tomorrow: drive-through COVID testing; telemedicine from my dining room table; keep hands washed; wear mask outside condo; keep my distance; drive-through dinner; early to bed.

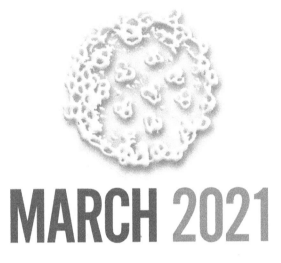

MARCH 2021

I've Got You Under My Skin

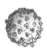

WEDNESDAY | MARCH 3, 2021

'M GRUMPY TONIGHT AND I KNOW WHY.

It's due to the unending public health idiocies being foisted upon us by conservative Southern governors who, despite all scientific evidence to the contrary, are busy abolishing mask mandates and social distancing requirements. Alabama hasn't joined the parade yet but our governor has a press conference set for tomorrow morning, and I'm pretty sure I can predict the substance of it.

This pisses me off for a couple of reasons.

First, while numbers are down and vaccines are rolling out, we are not out of the woods yet. The rapid spread of more infectious variants means that relaxing public health measures is likely to send us toward another surge. Every time we surge and numbers go up unnecessarily, for every thousand positive tests, three people receive a death sentence.

Second, it's also a huge slap in the face for an exhausted health-care workforce. The people they are going to have to take care of are going to be middle-aged folk who have either been unable to obtain a vaccine or who have been taught by their information sources that they don't need one. The elderly, being in the early group to get vaccines, will be relatively protected; the rapid decline in cases and deaths recently has been due to that low-hanging fruit having been plucked.

Then there are my purely selfish reasons. If we start surging again and it prevents me from being able to do my planned travel and get back on stage again, Imma gonna be mad!

I wrote an essay a couple of weeks ago for an elder care website. Rather than go stream-of-consciousness, I'm going to publish it here so I can spend the evening with my can of hard pear cider and old episodes of *Community*. Enjoy.

Why Can't I Find a Geriatrician For Mom?

Most human beings, as they age, realize that their bodies and physiology change from what they were in their younger adulthood. Things that never bothered them in the past start to hurt. Their reaction times slow. They have less strength and muscle mass. Eyesight and hearing aren't as keen.

American medicine began to understand that the precepts of medical treatment that were being developed post-World War II, full of a newfound scientific rigor, might not be one size fits all. For example, such specialties as pediatrics for children and obstetrics and gynecology for women were given new status.

Geriatrics, a specialty dealing with aging and the older adult, was first formalized in this country with the founding of the American Geriatrics Society in 1942. But there wasn't a lot of interest from either the medical community or from society at large as the number of individuals living healthy lives into their 80s and 90s was very small. Most people were carried off by acute illness somewhere in what we would now consider late middle age.

Things began to change in the mid-1960s.

First, the financing of health care for older individuals was radically transformed with the introduction of Medicare in 1965. This federal program, which was available to a majority of seniors, was instantly popular as aging adults suddenly had a resource for paying physician and hospital bills that did not rely on their own pocketbooks. The older population signed up in droves and by the early 1970s, Medicare was fully enshrined in our culture as an entitlement, becoming one of those third rails of American politics.

Second, demographers recognized and began to publicize what had been going on in America in the years following the end of the war. The relative privation of the Depression and World War II years, 15 long years of never enough, had given way to prosperity and a resulting dramatic rise in the birth rate from the mid-40s through the mid-60s, forever known to history as the Baby Boom.

The scale of the Boom was enormous. Society, rebuilding itself after years of trauma, was determined that this generation should never know want or unhappiness. A new media culture was created to reflect an idealized society from *Sally, Dick, and Jane* to *Leave It to Beaver.* Schools were built and enlarged. Public universities were lavishly funded to allow for their education at low prices. Their sheer numbers forced society to bend to their needs as they entered each stage of life.

><&=

Demographers, forever thinking of the future, projected forward and began to wonder about what this might mean when Boomers began to enter their elder years early in the 21st century, especially when other world populations were exploding, meaning more and more competition for resources.

The Boom itself, as it matured, tended to ignore these calls as they, to this day, consider themselves a young and vital generation. Those born in the first year of the Boom, turning 75 this year, contain such luminaries as Dolly Parton, Sylvester Stallone, Susan Sarandon, Bill Clinton, Sally Field, Donald Trump, and Cher—not exactly what we would consider a decrepit and over the hill cohort.

The medical system did start to take notice of what was coming and, in the early 1980s, began to formalize geriatric medicine as a specialty, creating (with the assistance of Medicare) specialized teaching programs for those who had completed initial training in either Internal Medicine or Family Practice.

These fellowships began to pop up in university training programs by the late 1980s, usually as subunits of other programs rather than as fully funded entities in and of themselves. Formal educational criteria were set and board exams were created to determine who had the necessary skills to be called a geriatrician.

For the first ten years of the board exams (mid-80s through mid-90s), there were two paths to becoming certified. You could either complete fellowship training or, if you had clinical experience in the field, you could apply to take the test based on that experience. Most individuals working in the field took the tests based on these grandfathering rules, and the number of board-certified geriatricians in the country rapidly rose, peaking at about 9,000 in the late 1990s.

Board certification is not lifelong; you must retest every ten years. Many of these early people who grandfathered in retired or found that maintaining certification was not worth the time and expense. Thus, the number of geriatricians began to fall. It's between 5,000 and 6,000 today.

Those who study medical systems and the impact of aging populations on them understand the role of the geriatrician in health care. Not everyone needs a geriatrician starting on their 65th birthday. Geriatricians are most valuable taking care of that subset of older people who have developed chronic disease burden to the point where their physical and/or cognitive function is impaired and they can no longer live independently in the life they have designed for themselves.

Most of these people do not live in nursing homes or other congregate facilities. They mainly live in the community, cared for by an army of family members and friends doing the best they can.

⤜•⤏

A geriatrician's special skills in understanding the interplay between social and physical determinants of disease, medication management, fall prevention, maintenance of continence, management of dementia behaviors, and other such issues can make the difference between a happy home life and misery for all concerned.

Medical demographers have concluded that by 2030, when this country will enter peak age (the entire Boom over the age of 65 but not yet having begun to die off in significant numbers), it will take about 30,000 geriatricians to provide optimal care— five times as many as are available.

We are still training new geriatricians. There are roughly 400 training slots available nationally on an annual basis. Only about 200 of them fill with applicants after the matching process is complete. Here at UAB, we have been unable to attract a single applicant for the last three years. At that rate, it would take well over a century to create the number we need in just a few short years.

Geriatric medicine is the second least popular specialty among US medical school graduates, bested only by geriatric psychiatry. The reasons for this are complex. Some are buried deep within the culture of the US medical education system that devalues person-to-person work relative to complex procedural work. Some are tied up in the financing of health care and the pivot by health systems away from unprofitable service lines. Some are due to the economics of physician compensation. Geriatrics remains one of the lower-paid specialties due to its reliance on Medicare reimbursement which is notoriously stingy for cognitive services.

This leads to a fundamental problem.

We have a rising demand due to the pressures from an aging Baby Boom on the health system. We have a society that has moved away from investment in public health infrastructure which would allow a less profitable specialty to sustain itself and provide compensation packages that would attract more medical graduates into the specialty. We have a stagnant number of qualified geriatricians. The 200 new graduates a year barely offsets the number who leave the specialty through retirement or change of job focus.

Those few of us who remain in the field and committed to clinical geriatrics are well aware of all of these trends and saddle up for work every day determined to do the best we can. The end result of all of this is that finding a geriatrician for Mom is exceedingly difficult. They just don't exist.

Can this problem be fixed in the short amount of time remaining before peak age? Of course it can. We know this from looking at recent medical history.

Prior to the 1990s, there was really no such thing as a hospitalist. There are now more than 40,000 of them nationwide. Financial incentives, working conditions, and system structures were changed in that decade to make it a viable choice for new physicians, and they came flocking to the job opportunities.

Something similar could be done for geriatric medicine. All it requires is a health system willing to make those changes, either intrinsically which would require economic inducements, or extrinsically through legislative fiat. These are things I cannot accomplish on my own. It will require societal will. In the meantime, I'll keep saving the world one patient at a time.

SUNDAY | MARCH 7, 2021

I'S SUNDAY EVENING.

I'm not in a foul mood. I really don't care what the Duke and Duchess of Sussex have to say about the British Royal Family. I've been able to scratch my theatrical itch.

The weather has been nice. Vaccination news has been incredibly positive with several million more people receiving their jabs in this country over the weekend.

><~@

So what to write about this evening?

Yesterday was about chores: bi-weekly grocery run; once-every-few-month Costco run; pet store for a big-bag-of-Science-Diet-Hairball-Control-Formula run; followed by laundry; reorganizing a number of things around the condo that had fallen into disarray; plus stowing away my makeshift film studio out of the dining room as *Tartuffe* is over and nothing else is on the horizon other than the filming of a lecture on basic geriatrics for a national board review course next week.

The next theatrical project, *The Pirates of Penzance,* is rehearsing and performing in person over the next five weeks—masks, social distancing, and all such other safety protocols in place.

Today was about connection. Online church service in the morning, picnicking in the park with old theater friends (properly socially distanced) in the afternoon, and the monthly extended family Zoom meet-up in the evening where the cousins all catch up with each other.

So I suppose the big questions I'm grappling with as things improve are: How much, how fast? What will be restored to pre-COVID norms? And what will remain altered?

><~@

We have certainly improved in terms of hospitalization and death numbers from where we were early in the year. The fall has been relatively rapid, likely due to the use of vaccines among the most vulnerable populations. However, vaccines are still coming online in fits and starts due to the previous administration's not putting the full force of the federal government's powers behind it and the current administration's need to play catch up.

We need to keep up all of our good habits for a while longer. If the amount of vaccine promised materializes, we'll be in a situation around Easter where the majority of people who have been chasing vaccines will have received them and we will start to see vaccines chasing people as the public health system tries to find harder-to-reach-and-educate populations.

A significant number of these people will need to be vaccinated in order for us to forgo masks and social distancing, otherwise, there will be large populations trading virus around and higher chances for mutations and reintroduction into more protected areas of society.

When can we have blow-out indoor parties and rehearsals and theater and sporting events and dances and all the other things we have been missing for the past year? I don't know. I'm hopeful for the fall, but a lot is going to depend on whether people who have been fighting against basic public health measures for political reasons come back into the fold.

>◉

I would keep an eye on Texas.

Their decision to completely open up everything as of this weekend will cause changes in behavior. Those changes in behavior show up as changes in case rates in 2-3 weeks, changes in hospitalizations in 4-6 weeks, and death rates in 6-10 weeks.

It will be interesting to see what happens in Texas in April in comparison to other states playing it safely. It will also be interesting to see if new mutations spread within Texas, and then beyond its borders as traveling Texans carry it around. With luck, none of these will cause serious issues, but one never knows, does one?

My professional life will have significant changes no matter what. Telemedicine is here to stay. I don't particularly care for it on my end as I feel like I miss far too much not being in the physical presence of my patient and able to pick up on subtle cues. It will be OK for what I call my "Well Baby Checks" on long-term patients with stable issues, as long as they come in person occasionally, but it's not good for new or unstable patients at all.

I also have a feeling that masks are likely to remain *de rigueur* in healthcare facilities long after the pandemic has faded. They've made such a huge difference in the transmission of viral illness in general, as evidenced by our essentially non-existent flu season, that the Joint Commission is likely to require them on staff (and possibly on patients). I wonder if we will adopt, in Western society, the habit of Asian societies of putting on a mask to go out when you have any sort of viral symptoms now that we've normalized them over the last year.

~⊱⊰~

Both my friend and family gatherings today were interesting as the focus was not so much on the past and loss, but on the future and what possibilities are to come. The theater friends were full of discussion about what would be needed to jump-start and rebuild live theater after the great pause. The family Zoom was about what was coming up with professional endeavors and future plans for pushing ahead with life.

I find this very hopeful.

Americans are incredibly resilient when we need to be. We move forward relatively well when given a few guideposts (and for the first time in years, I feel like we've been getting some from the very top). I only fear that as things improve and we all work on moving forward that we will forget the lessons the last year has taught us regarding work/life balance, how to care for each other as communities, how to listen to those of differing experiences, and how to slow down and savor smaller things.

I, for one, want to figure out a new balance between work, theater, writing, and just plain living. I don't know what it's going to be yet but going back to what was doesn't feel right. Forward, always forward—but with a mask on and social distancing for a few more months at least.

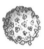

THURSDAY | MARCH 11, 2021

ONE YEAR: 525,600 MINUTES as Jonathan Larson taught us in his anthem from *Rent*.

One year ago today, the World Health Organization officially classified COVID-19 as a pandemic, and the coronavirus crystallized into the national consciousness in a way that it had not in the past. I had seen it coming. I know enough about virology and epidemiology from a physician's training to know it was out of control and coming our way several weeks earlier.

Näive as I was, I assumed that the combination of the resources of the US government and our national character of pulling together in adversity were going to help us brace for the impact and deflect the damage. I didn't understand just how hollowed out and damaged our institutions had become or how fractured we were as a society until those first few weeks when a combination of willfulness, ignorance, and spite took over what should have been a time of courage and sacrifice, laying the groundwork for the next year of our lives that would profoundly affect us all.

I had written the first piece of what was to become these *Accidental Plague Diaries* the evening before the WHO declaration. I was well aware of the issues and what was happening, but I was afraid to write about it, to actually give it form and shape with my words and make it more real. Eventually, the shadow on the horizon loomed too large.

There was no way I could not write about it and still make sense of the world. And so I wrote, and wrote, and wrote.

><><

On that day a year ago, there were a total of 29 known COVID deaths in the USA. As of today, there are nearly 531,000—roughly the same number as the number of minutes in Jonathan Larson's famous lyric.

If this mathematical reality hasn't hit you yet, let it sink in now. We've lost an average of one person a minute every minute for a year; one person a minute suddenly gone, leaving a hole in our social fabric and a bereft group of family and friends wondering why?

Pandemics are not new. They crop up routinely like other natural disasters such as earthquakes or hurricanes and have done so since the human race decided that hanging out in groups was beneficial. The difference this time around was an ignoring of the pandemic for political reasons, leading to a death toll many times higher than it needed to be.

Today, numbers are down and vaccine is out, but the mortality rate remains about 1,500 a day nationwide. That's enough to cut a full year off American life expectancy—two and a half years for most American populations of color; less for white populations. COVID was the third-highest cause of death for 2020 bested only by heart disease and cancer.

The new administration is halfway to the hundred-day mark. It seems to have solved the problems of vaccine manufacture, so there should be plenty of doses in the pipeline over the next month. But it has not yet completely solved the issues of vaccine distribution.

The previous administration's plan of just distributing to state health departments, chronically underfunded institutions without much clinical infrastructure, turned out not to be the wisest of decisions. As new rules have been put in place, and vaccine is now sent to health systems accustomed to creating clinical programs, things are improving in the get-the-shots-in-the-arm department.

But we've still got quite a ways to go.

UAB is opening up a fifth mass vaccination site next week, and I am pretty certain that the backlog of older and at-risk people waiting for vaccinations will be cleared in our area by tax day. The VA, for all its faults as a clinical system, with access to supplies from federal channels, has done a heroic job getting its patients vaccinated. The local VA has now given at least one shot to more than 50% of its active patients.

There's been some good news on the vaccine front.

New numbers out this week show that the Johnson & Johnson vaccine, where earlier studies showed less efficacy post-vaccination than Moderna and Pfizer, is pretty much equally effective after six weeks. So it doesn't really matter which of the three you get. Six weeks after the initial inoculation, you're pretty well protected.

There's also new data out of Israel (the country which has done one of the best jobs in getting its entire population vaccinated) suggesting that all of the vaccines significantly lower transmission rates in addition to protecting the individual.

Pretty much all of the adult US population seeking vaccines should be well protected by late spring. Then comes the problem of trying to handle the significant portion of the population which will refuse for political or other reasons. As long as that sector of the population remains the size that it is, the virus is going to continue to be an issue. I don't have a solution for this one.

A number of people have approached me about getting vaccinations for frail elders bed-bound at home who cannot easily be gotten into cars for drive-through vaccination settings. It's a population near and dear to my heart, the people who made me realize that geriatric medicine was my calling, and around whom I have designed my career. I know what the problem is.

The legislation regarding COVID vaccines has the cost of the medication itself borne by the federal government. However, providers are allowed to charge an administration fee (waived by most programs currently) to cover their costs for supplies/labor, etc. Delivering vaccines to homes is a labor-intensive proposition. Even using the Johnson & Johnson vaccine that does not require the cold chain still means a skilled vaccinator has to go out and administer it.

As all of the vaccines are under emergency use protocols, there are things that must be done in terms of paperwork and patient monitoring that are not necessary with approved vaccines like flu shots. It will take 30-40 minutes per household to deliver shots and, with travel time, you might be able to get in ten visits a day per vaccinator.

No one has decided that they want to be the organization that is going to absorb these costs (with the exception of the VA locally) which is why it's just not available. The state doesn't have the money. Almost all health institutions are for-profit in some way and aren't going to want to take on a considerable unreimbursed cost. This will get solved eventually, but things are at a bit of an impasse.

Until all of these kinks can be worked out, even if you're vaccinated, you know what you still need to do. Wear your mask. Wash your hands. Keep your distance. Like we're doing on our imaginary beach in *The Pirates of Penzance*.

SUNDAY | MARCH 14, 2021

IT'S SUNDAY NIGHT, the first day of Daylight Savings Time. My body is having a hard time deciding how late it is.

I'm boycotting the Grammys. I still haven't forgiven them for giving song of the year to *Killing Me Softly With His Song* over *American Pie* in 1972, and it's time for my bi-weekly update of *The Accidental Plague Diaries*.

I have no idea what I'm going to write about this evening, but that hasn't stopped me in the past. Something usually starts to take place as I let my fingers run over the keyboard.

The weather has been lovely and spring-like here in Birmingham over the last few days. Sunshine. The pastels on the trees are bursting forth in their usual sequence: tulip magnolias two weeks ago, Bradford pears this last week; flowering plums and cherries; dogwoods; redbuds; and gobs of wisteria still to come.

It's my favorite time of year here. The flowers are lovely, it turns warm without being hot, and the humidity has not yet crept into town. I tell people that if they want to visit, late March through early May is the time to do it.

We're not out of the winter woods yet though. There's usually a cold snap that breaks our weather into a first and a second spring, and it's threatening to arrive this next week.

I'm just hoping for good weather the second week of April when we perform *The Pirates of Penzance* outdoors. The only other outdoor show I've done in town was *Twelfth Night* for Shakespeare in the Park—in August. That was miserably hot and sweaty. April is a much better choice for performing *plein d'air* in this climate.

There has been very good news on the COVID front.

The number of vaccines available nationally is greatly accelerating. Per the CDC, nearly 4.6 million people received a vaccine yesterday. That's up from the record 1.6 million people last weekend. At this rate, the administration's goal of getting every adult American a vaccine who wants one by the first of May is likely to be met.

If you haven't gotten yours yet, it's coming. Just stay on those lists. The percentage of people refusing a vaccine, mainly for political reasons, remains too high for the epidemiologist in me to be comfortable. I keep hoping a certain ex-president, who was vaccinated himself in January, will publicly call for the vaccine as a step of atonement, but I'm probably reaching too high.

The most concerning issue remains the mutation of the virus and the rise of variants. The majority are still covered by the extant vaccine although there are variants in South Africa and Brazil where this isn't as clear. The last thing we need is a resistant variant winging its way around the world just as we're starting to get our vaccination game together.

The Astra Zeneca vaccine (not yet approved in the US) was considered one of the major hopes for poorer nations as it was inexpensive to manufacture and easy to store. There are reports out of Scandinavia of a number of serious post-vaccine clotting disorders, and it has been pulled in Norway. If this turns out to be a real issue, there's going to be a problem. We tend to forget in the US that the pandemic is a global, not a local, issue. Solutions need to be global in order for transmission to cease.

We're heading into the Easter season. In my house growing up, Easter was big for the egg hunts. The first one I remember was shortly after we moved into the house in which I did most of my growing up.

I was three, nearly four, and still an only child when I came down on Easter morning and was upset because I could only find two eggs. I complained vociferously to my mother who told me that the Easter Bunny had determined that I was getting smarter, that eggs wouldn't be in plain sight anymore, and that I needed to be more diligent in my searching. I went back and figured out that the Easter Bunny had put eggs inside of things or behind books.

In Easters-to-come, we were often traveling, either out to the Washington coast or down to San Francisco to see my grandparents. Our family Easter Bunny was quite resourceful at creating egg hunts in cheap motels and vacant fields across the road from cheap motels.

I kept up egg hunts well into adulthood. I used to do them for Steve when we lived in Sacramento. At one point in the mid-80s when I was still in med school, I invented a game for an Easter brunch at a friend's house called "Dr. Jekyll and Easter Bunny" in which there was an egg hunt with good and bad eggs.

The object was to gather good eggs into your basket and slip the bad eggs into other people's baskets when they weren't looking. I can still remember a bunch of adults tearing around a backyard to the strains of Mendelssohn's Italian Symphony as the game got underway. I haven't done a good egg hunt in a while. I have a plan to remedy that this year.

In the meantime, onward with other projects, but always mask on, hands washed, and distanced—unless vaccinated and around small numbers of other vaccinated people according to the CDC.

THURSDAY | MARCH 18, 2021

'M GROWING CONCERNED.

Things had been going well in Covidland. The Biden administration, after promising 100 million doses of vaccine in its first 100 days of office, has managed to deliver that amount in 58 days. The numbers had at least plateaued locally, and there was a hope that if we could hold steady we might have a relatively normal summer.

Now numbers are surging in Europe, trends are up-ticking here in the US and in Alabama, and we may be heading into another season of pain. We're just about to hit 30 million total cases here in the US (nearly 10% of the population), and we continue to lose about 1,500 people a day.

We're not going to know how the vaccine push has mitigated virus effects for another month or so. It takes about six weeks from initial injection to full immunity no matter which of the three formulations is used. We've only had mass vaccination available for the last few weeks, so just how things will play out is unclear.

The current uptick in cases represents social action from mid-February when it started to become clear that cases were falling significantly, and probably comes from people beginning to relax their social distancing and mask-wearing due to the widespread dissemination of that information.

I'm not sure what's driving the surge in Europe which is leading to new rounds of lockdown. My insight into social attitudes there is not as good as it is here. And I'm really unclear about the political backlash against the AstraZeneca vaccine which had been a mainstay of their vaccination plan.

Yes, there have been a few issues of serious clotting disorders, but it's unclear if the vaccination is the cause. The rate is only a small percentage of the clotting issues known to be caused by most birth control pills, and there doesn't seem to be any great hue and cry to take them off the market

There seem to be some indications that the AstraZeneca vaccine, as a British product, is caught up in EU/Brexit politics. At least we're not the only advanced society putting political considerations before public health.

I'm still very worried about our various social institutions and that something major may still collapse under the strain. We're still not out of the woods with COVID by a long shot. It might not take much of a change to bring down the healthcare system or the stock market.

Systems failures aren't usually caused by a massive blow, but rather through the accumulation of small problems which are overlooked or not thought to be serious enough to warrant the cost and energy of repair. Eventually, the cumulative rot brings the whole thing down.

I use this sort of model often when teaching my patients and their families about falls. There aren't a lot of geriatric disease states that I can make much headway with. No cures for arthritis or chronic kidney disease, for example.

Fall prevention, however, brings a lot of bang for the buck. Young people don't think much about falling. Young bodies and nervous systems deal fine with it, but the older you get, the more likely it is that there's going to be serious harm. One of the ways in which you know you've gotten old is the reaction of others when you fall in public. If they laugh, you're young; if they rush over in concern, you're old.

Falls are a systems failure—the system that allows our bodies to be bipedal. Most mammals are not. Walking around on two feet is difficult and hard to balance correctly. It takes most of us four or so years of all-day, everyday practice to get it right.

To do it, we must learn to coordinate our vision, what the balance mechanism of the inner ear tells us about gravity, what the outside world tells us (which when we stand and walk comes to us solely through the soles of our feet), and what a couple of hundred muscles in our legs and back are up to. All of that information ascends our nervous system, is processed by our brain, and then new signals are sent to the musculature to constantly adjust.

As we age, brain processing slows, the speed at which signals travel through the nervous system to the brain and back again slows, vision dims, muscles diminish in size and strength, and then there are the disease processes that can interfere like neuropathy, arthritis, macular degeneration, and Parkinson's. The ability of the brain and body to work together to maintain balance becomes tenuous.

When a young person suddenly loses balance, such as a slip on the ice, a whole series of reflexes immediately go into play (the brain knows "fall = bad" on a very primitive level). There's the dance as the feet scrabble to find purchase and the weight shifts quickly on the legs to try and maintain an upright posture. If the brain knows it's going down, there's a quick roll to get the arms and hands down to brace the body against impact. All of this is instinctual. You don't think about it, you just do it. If the fall is serious, the most common fracture is the wrist as the hand and forearm take the impact.

In an older person, the neural slowing means that gravity takes over before those reflexes can fully be implemented; it's not possible to get the hands out in time. Older people, therefore, break hips, vertebrae, and their skulls—much more serious injuries. We start backing away from fall risks instinctively in middle age. At 20, we leap from rock to rock across a mountain stream. At 50, we look at the rocks, then walk downstream and across the bridge.

We can't always fix the intrinsic causes of falls, but we can do something about the extrinsic ones by helping older patients eliminate fall risks at home and working with them on their gait and balance, teaching them some basics like not carrying things up and down steps, making sure there is adequate light, and how to adjust posture more slowly to avoid dizzy spells.

One of the things that becomes necessary is the use of an external device to improve balance, the dreaded cane. I have learned over the years, especially with the aging Baby Boom, never to refer to these things as canes. Canes are for old and frail people.

Young and healthy people in their 70s need walking sticks, alpenstocks, trek poles, shepherd's crooks, or some other such device that connotes health and exercise. In about 15 years, I'm going to invest in a wizard's staff and a pointy hat for myself.

This is not a new dilemma.

We know this from Greek mythology and the legend of Oedipus. Long before he had difficulties with his parents, he was wandering in Egypt and ran across the Sphinx. Not the nicest of creatures, the Sphinx asked a riddle of travelers. If they answered correctly, they were allowed to pass; if not, they were torn limb from limb and tossed in the ditch.

When Oedipus met the Sphinx, the ditch was full of decaying bodies as the Sphinx had not yet been defeated. Oedipus, being a cocky young man, said hit me with your riddle, to which the Sphinx replied, "What walks on four legs in the morning, two legs at noon, and three legs in the evening?" Oedipus thought about it and replied, "A human. First, they crawl, then they walk, and then they need a staff."

This was, of course, the correct answer and he was allowed to pass. This story, which is three or four thousand years old, shows us that the need for assistance in ambulation as we grow older has always been there. We just like to pretend we're not the same people our forebears were.

Thus endeth the lesson in geriatric medicine for the day. Go forth in peace, but washeth thy hands, weareth thy mask, and keepeth thy distance.

MONDAY | MARCH 22, 2021

I T'S ANOTHER ONE OF THOSE bolt-upright-at-4:30 AM mornings.

I don't worry when this happens as I know it's perfectly normal at my age. My sleeping patterns are becoming a bit more erratic, in general. Some nights I'll sleep nine or ten hours, some five or six.

On those latter nights, my brain is trying to get me into the old patterns of first and second sleep that the human race discarded with the onset of shift work and the electric light but which our primitive brains remember all too well.

I know I'll be sleepy again around 6:30, just in time for my first alarm to go off rather than for me to snooze for a few more hours, so today is going to be a long day with double-clinic and rehearsal to follow.

One of the chief complaints of many of my patients is "I can't sleep."

On gentle probing, I usually find that they sleep just fine, they just don't sleep in the patterns they think they're entitled to. We all think we should slumber in a state of complete unconsciousness for somewhere between six and ten hours as that's what we all remember from our young adult days. Young brains are wired to do that, older brains not so much

We're all cro-magnons. For the tribe to survive, the older adults had to wake up at night, make sure the competing tribe wasn't sneaking over the hill, scare away the saber tooth tiger, and count the children while the younger adults slumbered to conserve their energies for the mammoth hunt. So older adults naturally sleep less deeply and are conditioned by evolution to have periods of wakefulness.

The private letters and diaries of pretty much anyone prior to the mid-19th century speak of first and second sleep in such a way that it was clear that this was the norm. Scholars and other intellectuals often did their best work in the wee hours between the two periods.

The invention of factories led to the invention of shift work which required that sleep be compressed. And then electric light separated our daily cycles from the cycles of the sun. The response in western society was to train everyone from infancy to have a single sleep period of roughly eight hours. This was further reinforced in the latter half of the 20th century by television programming schedules.

Now, the elder population, socialized by all of that, feel something is definitely amiss when they wake up at night just as their brains are designed to do, and off they troop to the pharmacy to load up on Unisom, Sominex, and Tylenol PM.

The problem with this is that the active ingredient in all over-the-counter sleep aids (with the exception of melatonin) is diphenhydramine, often known by its original trade name of Benadryl. It's a pretty benign drug in young adults, which is why it's been sold over the counter for decades. It'll make you slightly sleepy and clean up your runny nose while it's at it because it's also a fairly powerful antihistamine (its original use).

Unfortunately, it's also strongly anticholinergic (meaning that it blocks the action of the neural transmitter acetylcholine—a transmitter that's used in various ways in the brain, gut, and bladder). In older people, where their neural systems are already in trouble from other processes, this can spell disaster. Acetylcholine is the major neurotransmitter involved in memory processes, so blocking it can cause significant memory issues.

This is the mechanism by which Alzheimer's disease causes much of its havoc. I have "cured" more than one case of Alzheimer's by taking away the over-the-counter sleep aid. There's also some evidence that routine use of diphenhydramine by the elderly can actually cause the brain changes of Alzheimer's. Other side effects are constipation and urinary continence issues.

There are prescription sleep aids that are relatively safe for older people that can be used. I try not to. I try to get older people to understand and accept their own natural body rhythms. I'm fine with such tried and true methods as warm milk and chamomile tea, and I don't mind over-the-counter melatonin. It's a natural brain chemical involved in the sleep cycle.

I do use sleepers in the demented who become completely divorced from the clock and household routines. It's not about them, it's about the family who still need to keep to work and school schedules, and really need to sleep when grandma decides that 3 AM is the correct hour for practicing her accordion.

❧

So where are we in Covidland?

We're just about to hit 30 million diagnosed cases. For those of you playing along at home, we hit 10 million on November 9th and 20 million on January 1st, so the curve is not as steep as it was this winter, but it continues to inch inexorably up. Deaths are at 542,000 and are still somewhere between 1000 and 1500 daily.

As I write these numbers, which would have been unfathomable a year ago, I realize that I've become inured to them. They seem less immediate, less real. Is that because I've had my vaccination and am less worried about myself? Am I just burnt out? Is it that the media is moving on to other things and while COVID remains in the background, it's not front and center in the constant information stream that bombards us all on a daily basis?

The vaccines keep rolling out at a fast and furious rate. In Alabama, everyone over 55 and everyone with a chronic health condition is eligible as of today. A significant portion of the population will have this protection shortly. We'll have to wait a few months though to know what that really means in terms of viral spread.

><

The governor of Florida, who has spent most of the pandemic in a state of denial and cooking the books regarding COVID data, has been given a lot of good press recently and has been leading the charge for fully opening up. This has led to the traditional spring break crowds flocking to Florida beach towns.

Young people at the beach are, of course, doing what young people at the beach do much to the consternation of their elders. Will this lead to a new surge as they return to their college campuses and towns after exchanging microbes?

With luck, the more vulnerable back home will have been vaccinated and, therefore, will be less susceptible, so it won't be as bad as last year. We've all heard about the unrest in Miami Beach and the imposition of a curfew. Out of curiosity, I went looking for social media pictures of the beach in Fort Lauderdale and other beach towns to see if they looked similar. Yup, plenty of mingling unmasked young folk there, too. The difference is that Miami Beach is a traditional gathering place for young people of color suggesting that America's systemic racism is rearing its ugly head once again in terms of unequal treatment.

><

If you decide to go to the beach in the next few weeks, just remember it ain't over until it's over. Vaccines aren't fully protective until about six weeks after your first shot.

It remains unclear how much the vaccinated can contract and transmit. So wear your mask around other people, keep your hands washed, and plunk your beach towel down away from those you don't know.

THURSDAY | MARCH 25, 2021

I T'S TORNADO WEATHER.

The line of storms set to come over metro Birmingham today is significant enough that the National Weather Service put out a rare 5/5 warning for dangerous tornadoes in North/Central Alabama.

The first major storm hit my area about 45 minutes ago. As usual, the central Jones valley in which downtown, UAB, and my neighborhood are located, were fine.

There are reports of a major tornado having blasted through the southern suburbs. No reports yet on damage or injuries, but I can hear various emergency sirens as they head south down highway 280.

And now we wait.

UAB and the VA both shut down early. I'm doing the work I have left for the day from home, much to the confusion of the cats.

The weather has suspended the local vaccination sites as they tend to operate out of doors. Supplies of vaccine have gotten better and better over the course of the last few weeks, so they've been able to work at full capacity, and the number of vaccinated continues to rise steadily. The total percentage remains lower than I would hope due to the difficulties of reaching some communities for political reasons, some for trust reasons, and some for access reasons.

Alabama still hasn't come up with a mechanism for vaccinating the elderly who cannot easily leave their homes. I know it's a problem that's being worked on, and I hope there's money in the recent stimulus bill that the state health department can use to get one of the larger home health agencies with state-wide coverage to take the project on.

We hit 30 million confirmed cases today, not quite 10% of the pre-COVID US population. With 545,000 dead, our current mortality rate is about 1.8%. So, for every 60 people or so who are told today that they have the virus, one has been handed a death sentence.

After the huge push to get elders vaccinated, most of the deathly ill are between 30 and 60 and without a lot of health and functional problems. This is going to continue to happen as long as there are significant portions of the population who refuse to protect themselves.

If the disease were to remain in populations of willful ignorance, that would be one thing. However, that's not how viral infections work. It will keep circulating in susceptible populations, continuing to mutate into new strains and, if those new strains are not well covered by either vaccine or natural immunity, there will be new breakouts in protected populations, and there is no guarantee that one of those new strains won't be significantly more lethal.

The rain and thunder are beginning outside again. I just hope that today is not as bad as April 27, 2011, when a huge outbreak of tornadoes swept through a number of local towns, most notably Tuscaloosa, and dozens were killed.

Tommy and I were both home early that day due to the weather and were in the basement watching a movie, just in case. We weren't really paying attention to the weather news. We only realized how bad it was when our phones began ringing like crazy with people from out of state calling to check on us.

We had no damage. We didn't even lose power. But we found a number of pieces of debris on the top deck and the yard that had fallen from the sky: pieces of shingles, a carpet tack strip, some random pieces of what looked like someone's expense report.

❧

You can prepare for pandemics. They are one of the most reliable and predictable forms of natural disaster, having occurred every few generations since time immemorial. You can prepare for tornadoes by recognizing that they will come where certain climate conditions exist, but you can't predict exactly where and when they will strike.

City planners of the 18th and 19th centuries were pretty good at placing residential neighborhoods (especially those for the wealthy) in places relatively shielded from natural disasters. For instance, the two parts of New Orleans that didn't flood during Katrina were the French Quarter and the Garden District.

I've always liked living in older neighborhoods, designed around the pedestrian rather than the car. They're walkable. Things are close in. And they are well-protected.

When Steve and I bought our house in Sacramento, we bought close to Sutter's Fort, the one part of the central city that had never flooded. Sutter had had the good sense to ask the local natives that question before building. Here, tornadic activity always passes well north or well south of the central city where I have always lived.

❧

I read somewhere that one of the reasons adults become so nostalgic for their college years is that it is the only time in their adult lives that they live in close proximity to their neighbors in a walkable environment with lots of things to do nearby during plentiful leisure hours. Then they grow up, move to the suburbs where the combination of urban planning based around the automobile and the ideal of the detached and the separate single-family home predominates.

Cities were designed for millennia to conserve land and to have people live cheek by jowl. You became familiar with your neighbors' lives. You were in and out of each other's homes. You spent lots of time together in public space as you didn't have as much private space. Rich and poor mingled, and there was a social encouragement of empathy. Sounds a bit like a college campus.

Then came the most destructive invention of the 20th century.

Not the atomic bomb, but the internal combustion engine. It allowed us to grow apart, to live lives hidden from each other. As a result, the fabric of community and extended family frayed. We no longer saw the whole of the messy and complex lives of our friends and neighbors, only the projections of what they wanted us to see, a carefully curated public face with no complication of the less than ideal family lives that might be going on behind the closed doors of suburbia.

This trend has, of course, gotten a lot worse with social media. The end result has been a moving away from empathy and love thy neighbor to climbing the social ladder by monetizing thy neighbor which certainly explains a lot of what goes on with the prosperity gospel and conservative Christian denominations.

I'll stay out of the suburbs and exurbs for the richer tapestry of my quasi-urban small city life. I just have to remember that I still have to love my neighbor from a six-foot distance for a while longer.

TUESDAY | MARCH 30, 2021

THE NEWS FROM COVIDLAND IS DECIDEDLY MIXED.
I wish it wasn't. I wish I could say that we are definitely on a downhill slide and that this was all going to be over soon, but it's just not yet possible to do that.

The big push for vaccinations is certainly helping. Most of my patients have been able to at least begin their series, and there have been many heartwarming stories from them of finally being able to leave their homes unafraid—reunions with children and grandchildren, and the picking up of social activities for those who have been locked down in congregate living facilities.

It's still a minority of the population that's been able to access vaccines to date. It gets better all the time thanks to the efforts of the current administration, but it's going to be a while before everyone who could benefit receives the shot in their deltoid of choice.

On the negative side, the numbers are not looking good. The numbers of cases and the numbers of deaths have both been steadily rising over the last few weeks. I think it's too soon to say we're definitely in another surge, but it cannot be completely ruled out.

What's driving it? Likely a combination of factors: spring break, a general feeling that we're getting towards the finish line so we can relax, governors in more conservative states relaxing mask mandates and other public health measures due to political pressure, the spread of new variants.

The problems with this initial rise over the last couple of weeks might represent the early stages of exponential numbers and, within a month, if they continue to rise in that way, we may be right back where we were in January.

The scuttlebutt among those of us in health care who work the COVID wards is that there's a bit of a sea change in whom they are seeing. As the elders get their vaccines, the people who are arriving sick as snot, requiring ICU care, are skewing younger and younger. These are people in their 30s and 40s, otherwise healthy, who are devolving from cold symptoms to nonfunctional respiratory systems in a matter of days.

We still have a ways to go and it's too soon to put away your masks and your good habits developed over this last year of pain and loneliness. It's going to be some months yet before a vaccine can really roll out to the younger adult population and, while the chances of any one individual in that group getting extremely ill aren't great, the vast population means that the absolute number at risk remains high, and all of those illnesses and deaths remain preventable.

※

I'm not sure what to make of the current dissection of the response to COVID by the previous administration that's occupying the press. Anyone with some knowledge of epidemiology and infectious disease isn't in the least surprised by the current spate of breathless revelations. Those basic facts were there to be seen by those who looked: from the deliberate hiding and downplaying of deaths in the state of Florida at the behest of the governor, to the toadying at the highest levels of the CDC, to the political whims of the previous president.

I don't feel any particular sympathy toward any of the public figures currently being caught with their pants down over previous COVID responses. They all knew the truth. They all chose not to speak it for whatever reason at the time.

One of the chief problems at the moment remains the language we use to continue our framing and understanding of what is going on with COVID and public health. We use terms such as "war" and "battle." This anthropomorphizes the virus and we then start to presume that it has feeling and thought and strategy.

It doesn't.

It's just a virus, doing exactly what nature designed it to do—spread. Its spread doesn't depend on its behavior. It has none. Its spread depends entirely on our behavior. The current rise is likely caught up in our choices as individuals and as a society.

This leaves me, of course, as an educated individual, both in the ways of humans and the ways of viruses, in something of a quandary.

I too wish to be free of the proscriptions of this last year, and I am fully vaccinated. I have allowed myself a bit more leeway in terms of socialization with other vaccinated folk, and I'm not overly concerned about socially distanced outdoor activity (witness my participation in the COVID-compliant concert staging of highlights of *The Pirates of Penzance*) but I'm not willing to doff my mask, yell "Whee!", and dive into a mosh pit.

I want to be a good guardian of society and particularly my patients. At the same time, the subtle cues of society are those of "get back to normal" for both economic and social reasons. It's not normal yet. It may be more normal than a year ago, but it's not two years ago, and if we don't keep vigilant, it isn't going to be.

I wish our governor, who is allowing our mask mandate to expire a week from Friday, would continue to push it for just a few more months, but she won't for political reasons, and I get that. I'm going to keep mine at hand. I've gotten used to them. Besides, I have collected quite a few that are fashion accessories.

＞〇

I return to the field with my VA house calls starting next week. It will be interesting to see what messages of the current administration and public health policy will have penetrated rural Alabama. Until then, keep the mask, keep the hand hygiene, keep the distance.

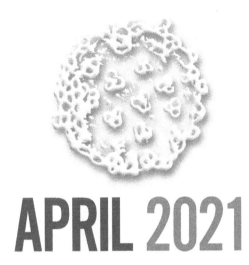

APRIL 2021

The Lost Liberty Blues

SATURDAY | APRIL 3, 2021

THERE'S A WEIRD DISCONNECT going on in my head at the moment.

Part of me is starting to believe that the pandemic is nearing an end, that things will continue to open up, that the US of four million vaccines administered a day and a rapid fall in cases from the highs of December and January will continue into a golden summer of everything is all right.

Then there's the part of me that looks at the data the media is downplaying.

The numbers of cases are roughly the same as they were during last summer's second surge; it just seems much lower coming after the huge numbers of this past winter. Mortality hasn't surged the way it has in the past. I assume this is because more cases are in younger and healthier people as vaccines have been distributed more widely among the elderly and the chronically ill, but I really don't know.

There are worrying trends from elsewhere around the globe. France and Italy are both going back into lockdown in certain areas due to spikes in cases. Brazil, thanks to the COVID denialism rampant in their executive branch, has a health system on the verge of total collapse.

More and more variants keep cropping up as large pools of unvaccinated individuals keep propagating the virus, giving it a chance to mutate. And a number of the variants appear to be more infectious than the original. None of them has yet proved to be more lethal, but there's a possibility that will happen. As long as a more lethal strain remains covered by the current vaccines, we will be OK.

Alabama's mask mandate expires on Friday and our governor will not renew it. I'm going to keep wearing mine, mandate or not, as it's still the right thing to do until the vast majority of the population has been vaccinated. At the rate we're going, that shouldn't take a whole lot longer.

I don't know what we're supposed to do about the portion of the population disinterested in being vaccinated for whatever reason. If it were a very small percentage of the population, it wouldn't matter as herd immunity would protect the group as a whole, but if it remains at the current level of 30% or so, that falls apart and all we have is a significant population which can keep reintroducing virus variants into the population at large.

Gaiety or gloom, which should I focus on? Both? Neither?

I'd prefer the former but I've been around too long to ever let the latter go unattended. Bad things are part and parcel of the world at large. Ignoring them doesn't make them go away. The gaiety side at the moment includes the CDC statement from late this week that it is safe for fully vaccinated individuals to travel domestically. I can now take my planned trip to Seattle free of guilt.

I'm still thinking of driving and making it a two-week road trip but I haven't completely made up my mind. I have Delta credits from plane fares for trips canceled by the pandemic which I could use instead.

Other happy things include *The Pirates of Penzance* which is coming together quite nicely. Masks make it hard to sing, and COVID safety protocols make the staging odd at best, but we've made it through six weeks together with no one getting sick. I can't say I'll look forward to rehearsing again in a parking garage, especially in an Alabama spring. Rehearsals have had ambient temps anywhere from the high 30s to the low 80s.

I was part of a Zoom reading tonight of a play retelling the story of Odysseus from Penelope's point of view. I played one of the vile suitors who eventually gets his comeuppance once Odysseus returns to Ithaca after his 20-year absence.

I'm hoping that some of this work that allows a cast to be gathered from around the country continues once the pandemic has passed. It allows performers to experiment in new ways which are rather freeing. The first half of *Tartuffe* I filmed has dropped, and if you've ever wanted to see me in a baroque wig. I rather enjoy classical theater. I hope I get to do more of it as live performance opens up again.

I'm trying to think of an amusing anecdote or other fun and pithy thing to write about as I finish up this entry in *The Accidental Plague Diaries,* but nothing comes to mind. Maybe I should do a few more columns on basic geriatric medicine. Perhaps I should go through my experiences and write down all the weird little things from my past I haven't yet shared. I'll take suggestions from the floor. On the other hand, I'll probably just continue to write whatever needs to come out.

WEDNESDAY | APRIL 7, 2021

HEARD ABOUT ANOTHER PHYSICIAN SUICIDE this morning. It wasn't someone I had ever met. I knew who he was from some of his postings in a group for gay male physicians. He was quick with a quip, had a nice sense of humor, and was posting his usual bad jokes up until the day he died. It made me wonder just what the mental health cost of this past year is really going to be, especially in medicine.

UAB gives us a little survey once a month to check up on our mental health. I have no idea what they do with the data they're collecting, but no one has ever called me concerned from the chair's office, so I figure they aren't overly interested as long as I keep showing up for work routinely—and vaguely on time. I could be a bit earlier in the mornings, but "not a morning person" doesn't even begin to cover it as anyone who has ever scheduled a 7 AM meeting with me can attest.

I'm not suicidal and am unlikely to ever be. All of the bad that's happened in my life, both personally and professionally, has given me a rather deep well of resilience that I draw on. I've been through the fire, survived, and it's going to take more than a viral pandemic and a societal shut down to really disturb my equanimity.

I'm also of an age where I know I'm looking at the end game of my career. I don't know how much longer I'll continue working. It's going to depend on a number of factors that are in constant motion. I have no intention of being in my 80s and tottering around the office older than my geriatric patients. I'm starting to get a few patients within a few years of me. That's scary enough.

I am worried about my younger colleagues.

They are giving up their 20s and early 30s to the educational treadmill, being forced into significant debt, and emerging into a health system that no longer truly values what a physician is. The corporatization of health care—and the changeover into a health industry that has shifted its goals from service and social mission to the manufacture of clinical encounters and hospitalizations for the purposes of profit— has resulted in a viewing of the physician as just one more cog in the machine.

The system recognizes that the physician is necessary. Laws dictate that nothing happens in the system without a physician's order. But the physician is not so necessary that he or she cannot be replaced with a less expensive adjunct, such as a physician's assistant, or second-guessed by sophisticated algorithms contained within information systems. More and more, physicians in their patient advocacy role are going to be slowly ground down by the implacable demands of the business side of the healthcare industry.

COVID has exposed many of the problems in the system for physicians. During the shutdown, when patients did not want to enter health facilities for fear of exposure, falling revenue streams led to cuts in salaries just as they were being asked to step up to the plate and bring their A-game to societal needs. The psychic strain on younger physicians caring for deathly ill COVID patients, many young and with whom they could identify, added additional burdens.

The current cadre of young physicians is too young to remember the HIV epidemic. I was in the thick of it. I sat at the bedside of many young men in the late 80s and early 90s. I held their hands as they died; there was no one else who would do it. Those of my generation have experiences we can draw on that younger ones don't.

The acute shortages of staff and the abrupt rise of telemedicine are leading hospitals to experiment with new ways of providing care that don't necessarily depend on patient and physician in a one-on-one setting. Better information systems are leading to the outsourcing of services to cheaper labor markets as in all other industries.

⤛⤜

I had predicted, decades ago, that the late 2020s and early 2030s were going to be a rough time for American medicine. This was based on demography and the aging of the Baby Boom. In 2030, we hit peak age with the oldest Boomers in their early 80s and the youngest just over 65.

However, I had not foreseen COVID and its effects on American health care which seem to have accelerated the negative trends so that we are in the midst of this transitional time now, a decade ahead of schedule. I can tell it has hit because the demands on me as a clinician from patients and families are accelerating.

The high levels of anxiety and depression engendered by the last year are starting to manifest in somatic ways and with people in constant need of reassurance. The paperwork load, with all of the transfer to telephonic and video conference services, has doubled.

People, now that they are vaccinated, are paying attention to body signals again in heightened ways and developing weird symptoms which need to be evaluated and followed up on. In an older person, there's always the question of whether something is a normal phenomenon falling within the ever-broadening bell curve or an unusual presentation of something which could be disastrous if missed.

One of the reasons I like being a geriatrician is that so much of our work is team-based. I don't always have to rely just on myself to stay on top of everything that could be wrong with my patients.

I'm human. I miss things all the time. But with competent nurses and social workers and pharmacists and therapists also looking at the picture, the missing puzzle piece is usually noticed by someone, and we can work together to craft a care plan that will ultimately help. When something goes awry, I often second guess myself and wonder what I could have missed or what I should have done differently.

When I was in residency and Steve and I were first together, I had a case like that where my patient died and I was kicking myself at home that evening assuming I had blown it in some way. The next day, at work, I opened up my backpack to find a rubber skull in it with a word balloon coming out of its mouth in Steve's writing saying "Dr. Andy, Why you kill me?"

That was Steve.

Quick switch of subjects.

The Pirates of Penzance has sold out. We had a spacing rehearsal in the amphitheater this evening and the show is going to work well. We are all now nervously watching weather reports as another storm/tornado front is due in the next couple of days. As long as it passes before Saturday at 2 PM, we should be OK, though we may have to do our dress rehearsals with umbrellas and gumboots.

I must say this was one of the easiest parts I've ever had to learn as the majority of my lyrics are variations of "Tarataratara" and I had those down at the first rehearsal.

COVID numbers are not looking good.

We added more than 450,000 new cases last week, and the British alpha variant has become dominant. It takes roughly six weeks between your first jab and attaining maximal immunity. People who have been vaccinated in the last month are still somewhat susceptible, and those beginning their series now won't be good to go until June.

Therefore, it remains imperative to keep up all those good habits. Wear your mask, wash your hands, keep your distance—even if you've had your vaccine.

SATURDAY | APRIL 10, 2021

TODAY IS TOMMY'S BIRTHDAY. He would be 56 if he were still living.

Perhaps it's fitting that I spent the day performing for his beloved Opera Birmingham in the inaugural performances of a shortened outdoor romp-in-the-park version of *The Pirates of Penzance*.

He was with me today. I could feel him running around the amphitheater, redecorating the set, supervising the front-of-house staff, and turning up in the pirate chorus.

Gilbert and Sullivan weren't really to his musical taste but he was all in on any project he had a hand in, whether he personally liked the material or not. He would even have appreciated the weather. Last night's thunderstorms dissipated by about 9 AM this morning; everything was sunny and cool by showtime.

Other than some minor bobbles with my police choreography in the second show (marching and singing in a mask is enough to make anyone tired), I felt it went well. The audience was more than appreciative to experience live entertainment conceived to be COVID-caution-compliant for both performers and spectators.

Many of the patrons were older. They've had their vaccines and are now venturing out after a year of confinement. The state's mandatory mask order expired yesterday. Our governor is not renewing it but is also not standing in the way of local ordinances or business decisions. Birmingham's mask order remains on the books a while longer and the audience was compliant without complaint.

Local numbers have been trending up again these last few weeks, mainly among younger unvaccinated folks. Jefferson County cases, which over the last two weeks had trended down from 80 to about 30 new cases a day, suddenly spiked at the end of last week to over 100 again, likely the result of spring break. Hopefully, it's a momentary spike and will immediately trend down again.

Total US cases keep going up.

We're over 31 million diagnoses now with more than 561,000 deaths. Only about 60,000 more to go until COVID surpasses the Civil War death toll —and that took four years. On a more modern scale, the number of dead just surpassed the population of Albuquerque to become the 32nd largest city in the country.

I've been searching lately for a medical topic to write about.

Yesterday, one of my patients brought in some new patent "brain food" they've been taking to stave off the memory loss of aging. I always ask that people bring me the bottles of such things so I can scan the ingredients and determine if there's anything in them that might interfere with other medications or that might cause unpleasant side effects. Most of them are vitamin and mineral supplements (not harmful for the most part, but often not necessary) with various herbs added (potentially problematic depending on the blend and strength).

As a physician with a relatively holistic approach to health, especially with an aging population (most older people understand their bodies quite well, having lived in them a long time, and know what to do to keep them well balanced), I never discourage people from doing what they think is best for themselves. I just try to give them any information I have grounded in science so that they can make educated choices.

I have a local chiropractor I trust to whom I refer as they can sometimes be more helpful for low back pain than allopathic medicine. I also refer to an acupuncturist/herbalist locally. There's a local complementary medicine clinic run by a well-trained doctor who works effectively with the anxious and somatisizers and who is smart enough to refer back to me when he recognizes some real pathology. I don't see any of these as being any sort of problem for the right patient. So much of medicine is getting people to tap into their own body understanding and wellness. These are just additional tools to do that.

I'm not as fond of the pills.

Actual herbs and extracts used in traditional ways are fine but the lumping of a lot of things together, slapping a pretty label on it, and advertising it all over late-night television is something else. The manufacturers of such products who had long run riot selling pretty much anything in a bottle were brought to heel by the Dietary Supplement and Health Education Act of 1994.

This piece of legislation allows these products to be classified legally as nutritional supplements and therefore exempts them from regulation by the FDA as drugs. In return, they are not allowed to be promoted as a cure for any sort of disease, and the labels are, in theory, supposed to match what's actually in the bottle.

Multiple studies show that about 1/3 of these products do not contain what's listed on the label. Another 1/3 contain active ingredients which are not listed.

A 2013 study of supplements found over 750 varieties that contained unlisted pharmaceutical drugs which should be FDA regulated. That's why the ads always say things like "not intended to cure any disease." They are sold for vaguely defined conditions such as "wellness' or "more energy." I gently try to steer people away from them.

At the same time, I do recognize the desperation people feel when faced with serious illness in themselves or a loved one. I've felt it myself when confronted with two husbands critically ill with conditions for which I could offer nothing other than love and presence.

If I thought there was healing magic in a bottle available, I would have raced out and gotten it, no matter the obstacles. My training, however, makes me understand that miracles are rarely obtained in capsule form.

This wasn't always the case.

A couple of generations ago, in the depths of World War II, brilliant minds finally figured out what Alexander Fleming's orange mold penicillium was actually good for. When applied to injured battlefield troops, it prevented the wound infections and septic shock that had always killed the majority of soldiers.

The antibiotic era was born.

After the war ended and there was enough of the new wonder drug left over for the civilian population, previously fatal infections were beaten back. Mix this with an intact infrastructure (the only one in the Western World after World War II) and the idea of American exceptionalism in medicine was born. In the immediate post-war years, this was absolutely true.

The idea that miracles could be found in pills took full root in American culture and to this day, everyone wants a quick fix two-week course of something. While this model works fine for acute infectious disease in the young, it's not so helpful for the usual chronic diseases of the elderly.

The best thing is primary prevention, keeping disease from ever setting up shop in the first place. This usually requires an understanding of good health habits and a willingness to partake of them routinely. Most people would rather do what they want when they want and then demand a quick fix from the doctor when things have broken down enough to require serious intervention and repair.

This will not sit well with the Baby Boom in particular. They're going to be livid in another decade when they finally figure out that neither I nor any other physician in the country has a copy of Ponce de Leon's map tattooed on our hineys—and that we can't turn back time. (Sorry, Cher).

If you knew Tommy, give him a thought today. And have some carrot cake in his honor.

TUESDAY | APRIL 13, 2021

I T'S THE OTHER SIDE OF THE WEEKEND. That means it's
Steve's birthday today.

It was 20 years ago this evening that we had his last birthday
party. He'd be 73 were he still here, likely running around making art
and stirring up trouble wherever he could.

Steve loved birthday parties as much as he hated growing older.
We invited over the few friends we had made since moving to Birmingham, mainly church people, as a combination of culture shock
and his illness limited our socializing over the previous few years.

He wore our birthday shirt.

It was a shirt he had bought me for my birthday some ten years
before. He gave it to me, then decided he really liked it and declared
that he was taking it back. I wrapped it up and gave it to him for
Christmas. He gave it to me for my next birthday, and so on. I think it
was wrapped and unwrapped more than a dozen times over the years,
a standing joke between us until the end.

That's the hardest thing about losing your partner.

You lose the person with whom you've built a history of hundreds
of private jokes and pet moments. You want to say "Do you remember
when…" but the only person that could possibly answer that with a
"yes" is no longer there.

I suppose, in part, that's one of the things that's spurred me into
writing these pieces over the last few years. I want to keep remembering when, and this is one way to get those stories out to a new audience that might appreciate a few of them.

Most of my Birmingham friends never met Steve. He became ill
about a year after we arrived and before we had a chance to create

much of a social circle. He was gone before I returned to the world of the performing arts that I had left for medicine so many years prior.

I suppose the second week of April is always going to be a bit of a difficult time, as long as I live, due to the proximity of Steve and Tommy's birthdays. Note to self: Try not to plan anything too emotionally involving for that week going forward.

Fortunately, *The Pirates of Penzance* is not Ibsen or Arthur Miller. And it is now over, to be replaced eventually with whatever the next theatrical project shall be.

There's nothing on the horizon yet, but I'm not worried. Something's bound to come along for the summer as things continue to open up.

Perhaps this is the summer to revive Shakespeare in the Park. I've only done that once and, as much as I enjoyed it, outdoor theater in Birmingham in August is not overly pleasant for either cast or audience due to certain peculiarities of climate.

I still have great hopes for summer, despite today's not-so-great news about the Johnson & Johnson vaccine.

A couple of things everyone should keep in mind: (1) Correlation is not causation. Just because two things happen together in time does not mean that they are linked; and (2) The number of reported cases of clotting is very small (six out of 7 million doses of vaccine administered).

All case reports involved women between 18 and 48. The background incidence of significant clots in women of this age isn't all that different. Women are more prone to clots than men as estrogens are thrombotic in nature. About 0.3% of users of oral contraceptives develop clots because of this. Other risk factors include smoking and being sedentary, and we know nothing about how any of these may have played into this cluster of cases.

If you've received the Johnson & Johnson vaccine, don't panic, even if you're a woman under 50. The chance of you having a problem is about the same as being struck by lightning.

If you were scheduled to get it and your appointment has been canceled, don't panic. There's plenty of Pfizer and Moderna in the pipeline to make up the shortfall. The system has figured out how to get vaccine into people in record numbers over the last month with between four and five million shots happening daily.

My biggest fear in all of this is that the media, who long ago abandoned in-depth reportage and nuance for sensationalism and clickbait, will write a lot of misleading headlines that will push people on the fence away from vaccination. If we're going to return to a sense of normalcy, we need as many people immune as possible, whether from immunization or from having had the disease—something I wouldn't wish on anyone as even mild cases seem to have significant issues with cardiac and nervous system inflammation that have unknown long term consequences.

Alabama may have abandoned its mask mandate, but the city of Birmingham has not. We were doing really well the last few weeks with one of the lowest levels of transmission in the country (only Arkansas had better numbers). It will be interesting to see if the dropping of the mask mandate by the state will start leading to an increase around the end of the month. I'm still wearing mine. I've gotten used to the thing— other than when trying to march and sing at the same time.

The British alpha variant has, as predicted, now become the predominant strain in this country which is a problem given that it's significantly more transmissible than the original strains. The patterns in high transmission states such as Michigan show that it is spreading rapidly in young, unvaccinated populations.

The majority of those folk, being healthy, will weather the storm, but there are more and more 30- and 40-somethings being admitted to hospitals in dire straits with no prior significant health history. These are people who don't need to die if we will continue to toe the line a while longer.

So wear your mask in public, even if no one else does. It sets a good example. Keep your hands washed. Get your vaccine.

SATURDAY | APRIL 17, 2021

'VE BEEN EXHAUSTED THIS WEEK, tired to the point of forgetting to set my alarm yesterday and waking up 20 minutes after I should have been at work.

I proved that I can be in a patient room within 15 minutes of opening my eyes. And I was able to get my schedule back on track. But I haven't done anything like that in years.

Usually, on mornings when I don't have to get up, I wake up within about 20 minutes of my usual alarm time, and then, when I realize I can sleep in, I roll over and go back to sleep for a while longer.

The weariness this week, however, has been bone-deep. I have little on my schedule over the next few weeks other than usual work things, so I'm going to listen to my body and try to unwind.

We passed 3,000,000 COVID deaths worldwide this weekend.

The US total continues to inch up as well and is now at 567,000. It's not racing upwards as badly as it could, probably because new cases are more likely to occur in healthier and younger individuals, older populations being more likely to have received vaccines at this point.

It wouldn't be so bad if the US character regarding health care weren't out in full force. We've more or less decided as a society to allow the vaccine to do all the heavy lifting for us so we can all get back to our usual lives.

The current administration has done a phenomenal job of getting the vaccine out. Half of US adults have now had at least one dose. Somewhere between three and five million jabs are happening daily.

US culture has always had a quick-fix mentality when it comes to health care. People come to us, as healers, expecting that a pill or a shot will take care of what ails them. While this may be true of common infectious diseases of the young, it's certainly not true of the disease processes of aging and body neglect such as diabetes or atherosclerosis.

Successful treatment of these generally requires lifestyle modification, prudence, and moderation in regard to such things as diet, exercise, and sleep, along with a willingness to partner with we physicians for the long haul. Most Americans have difficulties with these concepts.

Successful primary care physicians, like myself, have to figure out where the boundaries are between what we can control and help with, and what are the responsibilities of patients and their family systems. Those who don't negotiate that tightrope successfully generally don't do well with ambulatory care. It's difficult, and most doctors who work with inpatients have, at best, a limited understanding of it. Unfortunately, it's the inpatient docs who have political clout and the ear of administrators.

It takes roughly six weeks from the first shot—no matter which version you get—until you develop full immunity. Shot one, then shot two, three or four weeks later, then two more weeks until full immunity develops for Pfizer and Moderna; six weeks after the single shot for Johnson & Johnson.

Six weeks ago, we were in early March. Vaccine was just beginning to become more widely available after having been reserved for healthcare workers and at-risk seniors. The people given vaccine in the first week of March have only just become fully immune. Everyone who has received vaccine after that isn't there yet, and we've only really opened up the vaccine lines to all comers in the last week or so.

We're not going to have significant population immunity until Memorial Day. This is why it's so important to continue to wear masks indoors with other people and to keep up the social distancing. We've still got a ways to go.

The vaccine isn't 100% effective.

There have been roughly 5,800 COVID cases in the US in individuals who were previously vaccinated. When you divide that out over the 125 million of us who have been shot up so far, it's a very small number. The majority of the cases have been mild, but 78 of those 5,800 died of the disease.

Don't let all those good habits built up over the last year go to waste yet. It's going to take a combination of the vaccine and proper social behavior to restore things back to a semblance of normal—not just vaccine alone.

><()>

There are very few quick fixes in medicine outside of antibiotics and some surgeries. Sometimes, the fixes are unique, idiosyncratic, and dependent on the individual. I learned long ago never to argue with success when it came to my patients.

Some years back, an elderly man came to see me. He had an obvious dementia to which he and his family were somewhat oblivious. Even when the family had taken him for his driver's license renewal, and the examiners insisted on a road test, and the first thing he did was drive the car into a dumpster, none of them was willing to admit that perhaps his mentation had changed in his 90 years.

When I asked him why he had come to see me, he told me it was because someone had replaced his nose with a metal valve and he was afraid that when he slept at night, someone was going to close it off and then he would die.

I sympathized with his plight and asked him how he might prevent that. "Oh, I have a sure-fire way," he said. "Before I go to bed, I wrap a plastic bag around my head and then rubber band a washcloth over it. Then I put two scoops of vanilla ice cream on the washcloth, put on a stocking cap, and go to bed. Works like a charm."

I was a bit taken aback. The only follow-up question I could think of was, "Does it have to be vanilla? Will other flavors work as well?" He was so pleased with himself that I let him and his family work all of that out—including the laundry.

Today was Prince Philip's funeral; he missed completing his hundredth year by only a few months. Her Majesty looked small and frail and alone. I expect her to go on for a few more years, but it's likely that her public schedule will be greatly reduced. My cousins, the Earl of Snowdon and Lady Sarah Chatto were among the cortege, looking decidedly middle-aged. I guess that means none of us is young anymore. (Their paternal grandmother and my maternal grandfather were cousins. I've never met them, never will. If you've ever seen *The Crown*, you'll know why.)

I wonder what will happen when the Queen dies? She's been on the throne for nearly 70 years. Few are left with adult memories of life under any other monarch. I expect the institution of the monarchy will survive. It's one of the things that makes Britain Britain.

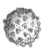

WEDNESDAY | APRIL 21, 2021

'M BACK TO NORMAL.

Or as normal as I ever get. I think I was born under an eccentric star and have been just a bit off-kilter ever since.

A number of long deep sleeps and a few naps have restored my equilibrium. I am back in my usual physical space of feeling just a little bit aged but with the ability to power through typical workdays with some leftover to expend on a project or two at night.

With nothing much theatrical coming up in the near future, it's time to tackle the bins of family papers, photographs, old theater programs, and other ephemera that have been staring at me from the front hallway since January. It will give me the excuse of scanning in a few more pieces of visual memorabilia to share with my stories.

My Facebook timeline is a plethora of vaccine selfies.

The full opening up of appointments for everyone over the age of 16 has been accomplished. This means that by Memorial Day, a significant portion of the healthy population will have received vaccine. By the Fourth of July, most of those wanting to be vaccinated will have finished their six weeks of marinating and will be good to go. I'm hopeful this means that the pandemic will be under reasonable control by fall and we can resume most normal activities.

There are two challenges that may hold this back.

The first challenge is that portion of the population holding on to political ideas about the virus and vaccination that are making them avoid getting their shots. If it was a small minority, it would be immaterial. That misunderstood concept of herd immunity would take over and protect society from significantly spreading coronavirus anyway.

But it's not a small minority.

Polls suggest it's more like 30% of the population. That's a large enough group to prevent eradication of the pandemic. It's also enough people to keep trading virus back and forth, setting up new strains which could potentially become more lethal or slip by vaccination rendering that immunity useless.

The second challenge is the usual American idea of exceptionalism keeping us from understanding that this is not a uniquely American problem. This is a global pandemic. It's everywhere from the concrete canyons of Manhattan, to the jungles of the Amazon, to the plains of central Asia.

We live in an interconnected world. Given modern travel technology, most of us are capable of reaching pretty much anywhere on the planet within 24-48 hours, and our microbes come along for the ride when we board that Airbus A-320.

To truly beat the pandemic, it has to be forced back not just here but everywhere. That means getting out billions of doses of vaccine, many to much poorer countries with sketchier transportation networks and less robust governmental institutions. With more stable leadership now in place, we can come together with other advanced countries and help with a worldwide concerted effort, but it's still going to take a bit of time, energy, and money.

While the pandemic is coming under control domestically, cases here in Alabama are up about 10% over two weeks ago. The absolute number looks pretty good, about a tenth of what it was at the peak of the winter surge in January, but any uptick is worrisome. It's probably the result of spring break, the governor's letting the mask mandate expire, and a general movement of people back into public space as vaccines take hold.

Anecdotally, most of the people being admitted currently are young/middle-aged, and the mortality rate isn't quite as high. But a number of them remain extremely ill so please, everyone, don't fall off the horse right before the finish line. Keep up those good habits until six weeks after your initial vaccination and beyond to protect your neighbors who are behind you in the line.

The global picture, however, is not so good.

There were more new cases of COVID worldwide last week than in any week since the beginning of the pandemic. Numbers are pushing upward in Brazil, India, and Southern Africa due to more infectious (and in some cases more lethal) variants.

They will get here eventually. It's inevitable. But, with luck, we'll have enough vaccine out there to keep them from getting a significant foothold in the population, and our reinvigorated public health institutions will be able to identify and isolate them quickly, as should have been done last year.

>——∘

I had a recurring dream with all my weekend napping. I re-enrolled at Stanford and decided to start anew on my college career. But I was trying to do it with my nearly 60-year-old brain, and I was floundering and failing and having a fairly rotten time.

None of my classes was meeting where it was supposed to. The layout of the campus kept changing. The bursar's office was dunning me for tuition bills for courses I was pretty sure I hadn't taken (History of Roman Chariot Racing? Advanced Bipolar Disorder?) After the third time, I found myself back in the same general milieu, I was ready to give up on higher education.

I woke up wondering what my subconscious was trying to tell me. Was it a Groundhog Day phenomenon born of this incessant pause in living patterns? Had I sniffed a madeleine before falling asleep? Was I trying to recover lost youth? Perhaps my brain knows I'm approaching a crossroads and is warning me not to take the same old road, but to veer onto some other path in the yellow wood.

Seven more work days until I have a chance to try and clear the brain and the plague diary morphs, at least in part, into a travel diary for a while. In the meantime: wash your hands; wear your mask indoors around people you don't know; and stay out of the mosh pit until at least six weeks after your initial vaccine.

SUNDAY | APRIL 25, 2021

'M RUNNING ON EMPTY.

Fortunately, I have only five more days until I get my time off and can recharge the batteries. One of the major reasons I decided to turn this into a road trip was a chance to disconnect from my usual world for a while. The nature of my job and career is such that there are lots and lots of people out there who rely on me for succor and counsel and empathy.

I have a lot to give but every one of those encounters leads me to give away a bit of myself and my energy. Eventually, the well starts to feel like it's running dry. A couple of weeks without feeling like everyone wants a piece and I will hopefully start feeling a little more in balance.

Tonight is the Oscars. I'm not watching.

This pandemic year has upended my usual moviegoing habits. I've seen none of the films up for the big awards. There are a few on my radar which I should catch streaming on one service or another eventually. The theaters are starting to open up again, but I don't think I'll feel comfortable going in to sit among strangers with my overpriced bucket of popcorn and soft drink for a while longer yet.

I've been watching more long-form television than film recently. This seems to be where all the good writers have drifted to, and it comes in easily digestible chunks between work projects, writing projects, and keeping things up on the home front in the evenings.

There are plenty of older films out there to keep me going when I truly want a movie. Will I be able to go to the movies again? I'm sure I will. But I can't imagine feeling safe prior to the fall, and even that is going to depend on what happens with COVID numbers and with all of the ramifications of the never-ending politics of vaccines.

The big hotspot at the moment in Covidland is India, likely driven by variants that are more highly infectious, although the authorities are still trying to figure out why cases, beaten back over the winter and early spring, started to skyrocket over the last few weeks.

There's so much that we still don't know about this disease, its pathology, and its epidemiology. Apparently, last month was election season in India with Prime Minister Modi and other politicians addressing huge crowds. As usual, the virus exploited a change in human behavior patterns to its advantage.

There is one variant in India, dubbed Delta by the WHO, that has the health authorities concerned. It has changes in spike proteins that allow it to bind more tightly to human host cells, making it significantly more infectious. If this variant combines with the ones originating in Britain that make it more transmissible person to person, we may have cause for alarm. I have a trip planned for India in the spring of 2022. I shall, as always, be cautious.

This week marks the third anniversary of Tommy's death.

I know it's time to move on, and in many ways I have, but the pandemic nature of our lives keeps me cocooned away from the world when I'm not at work. I'm getting better about going out than I was a few months ago. But seeing people socially still seems awkward and forced. It's as if the usual rules of etiquette have been suspended, and we're all feeling our way together into new patterns of being with others who are not of one's immediate family circle.

Handshakes and hugs are still *verboten*. Subjects to talk about are limited when no one has done much over the last year. I feel like I need to take a lesson from Eliza Doolittle and stick to two subjects: the weather and everyone's health.

So if you hear me asking about a new straw hat that should have come to me, you'll know the reason. I've been told the next of the Zoom theater projects is *Pygmalion* with me as Colonel Pickering, so I may be picking up a few Shavian epigrams in the coming months.

I had Hope, the Red Prius, serviced and detailed this weekend, making sure she was ready to drive 6,000 or so miles the next few weeks. The folks at Hoover Toyota told me that all was well so, if the pistons fall out in the middle of South Dakota, you know whom I will be calling on the Gods of the Lakota to strike down in vengeance.

I've downloaded some decent books to the Audible account, and I've mapped out at least four different routes. Having driven across the country a half dozen times, I've seen a good deal of it, so which route I take is likely to depend on weather patterns, snow reports, and my mood of the morning after downing a caramel macchiato from the closest Starbucks.

Now I just have to pack a few necessities (travel was easier before my dependence on CPAP which takes up a third of a suitcase) and find my decent sunglasses. Yes, I will write my usual travelogues. But I need something to write along with them: Family stories? COVID updates? Discussions of aging and health topics? A bit of all three?

I generally don't know what I'm going to write when I sit down to bang on the keys and produce these musings, but I do take requests.

Often, a comment or something someone says to me will inspire a topic.

The weather is lovely. Get out and enjoy it, as I did this afternoon with Opera Shots in the Opera Birmingham parking lot. The next one is Sunday, May 16th at Collins Bar downtown. That block of 2nd Avenue North will be closed, so get a drink and enjoy some good singing. I'm planning on returning from the road that day. Whether I turn up or not will depend on when I get back to town.

Enjoy your martini, but remember to social distance and keep your mask on around people you don't know. And grab some Opera Birmingham-branded hand sanitizer while you're there.

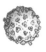

WEDNESDAY | APRIL 28, 2021

T'S APRIL 28TH AGAIN.

Another year has passed, and now Tommy has been gone for three.

I thought about going out to Parrish to put some flowers on his grave but other life chores intervened. I don't think he minds. He was never one for fuss, ceremony, and ritual unless it involved children and socializing them into the mysteries of the grown-up world.

Valentines? Anniversaries? Forget about it. He had no patience for Hallmark holidays. I once made the mistake of bringing him roses at work on our anniversary. He was not amused and let me know in no uncertain terms just what he thought of that gesture and my lack of imagination for executing it.

But, if a child or group of children of his acquaintance had something special that needed celebrating, he was all over that. While packing up the house this last year and moving, I found his stash of all-purpose child gifts. They're now being used by me for appropriate occasions over time.

⊷

Tommy and I didn't talk about death much. I think there were two reasons for that.

The first was the shadow of Steve that hung over our lives. As Steve was dead, he was both omnipresent and unknowable to Tommy. They never met. I did figure out later that Tommy had probably waited on Steve and me at the Eastwood Olive Garden a couple of times after we first moved to Birmingham, but neither Tommy nor I had any real memories of it. Talk of death with Tommy would, of course, rope Steve into the conversation, and that was a subject best left in the past.

The second reason was that Tommy had far too much living to do and way too many plans to let a nuisance like death get in his way. Even during that last hospitalization, he was working on wig designs and plots for his summer shows and trying to figure out how to go back to school again for yet another degree.

He was interested in seminary with an eye on a concentration in church music and hymnody. I found a few sketches for an idea for a musical setting of the Latin Mass in his papers. That would have been an interesting—and massive—project.

The one time I remember asking Tommy about what he would want in terms of arrangements should he die, he looked at me and said, "You'll have to figure it out; I won't be here," and went back to whatever he was working on.

Tommy's relatively quick decline and unexpected death were very different from my experience with Steve. With Steve, we had roughly two years from the time we learned he was seriously ill with his pul-

138

monary fibrosis until his passing. We both knew it was coming, made some basic arrangements, and then, never revisited the subject until it actually happened.

There was no need.

We lived our lives around his living, not his dying, and those two years were some of the best times we had in our 13 years together. Steve let go of the rat race of trying to be successful and make money, burying himself in his art, his garden, and his love of the little things. He was pretty much at peace, possibly for the first time in his life.

He had not had an easy existence as a younger man. He came out as gay in high school at age 14. That's not an uncommon story these days, but that was 1962, and his attitude from the beginning was to defy the world and anyone in it who would not accept him for exactly who he was.

He spent his 20s and 30s in Los Angeles, part of the avant-garde set around West Hollywood and Studio City, where he knew everyone and went to all the parties of the demimonde in the late 60s and 70s. He had all sorts of stories. The 80s and HIV destroyed his life and decimated his social circle and friendships, causing him to flee North to the Sacramento area to become his mother's caregiver after she was diagnosed with cancer, and that's where we met.

Between Tommy and Steve, I had nearly 30 years of partnership/marriage whatever term you want to use for it.

><s

I wrote a sermon a few years back, before the Obergefell decision, on the word "marriage" as applied to gay couples, and how our inexact language uses a single word in law for two radically different constructs: a civil contract that defines a family unit in the eyes of the state; and a sacred covenant that defines a union in the eyes of a church.

The pro-gay marriage forces were fighting for access to the contract. The anti-gay marriage forces were fighting to protect the covenant. They're still talking *at* each other rather than *to* each other, so I don't believe for a moment that this particular war is at an end.

I miss the coupled state, having been out of it now for three years, but I don't know if I want to do the work necessary to get back in.

Keeping a gay male relationship alive and solid is difficult. There aren't a lot of supports and foundations for it within either gay culture or straight culture. One believes that you should be free to find the next hot thing, the other believes that you're intruding on sacred ground in some sort of burlesque. This requires two men in union with each other to have to pour enormous resources in terms of emotional energy into the relationship and to be willing to make sacrifices to their socialized roles for the good of the unit. It's very hard.

I have nothing but admiration for my friends who have managed to do it over the years because I know just how much work they have to do behind closed doors. And I have nothing but sympathy for my other friends who can't overcome all of the obstacles and make it work over time.

I'm never going to say never in regards to a potential third husband, but I have no plans to start looking in the near future. There are a number of hoops any potential candidate would have to jump through. I know I'm not going to just settle to have someone in my life.

Maybe I'm a victim of Mona's Law from *Tales of the City* as defined by Armistead Maupin: "You can have a hot lover, a hot job, and a hot apartment, but you can't have all three at once." I've got the job and housing covered so the third might be asking a little too much of the universe at the moment. If I do find someone, going back to Mouse and *Tales of the City*, I just would like someone with whom I could buy a Christmas tree.

Sleep well, both Steve and Tommy, and know that I am forever richer and better for having been yours.

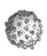

FRIDAY | APRIL 30, 2021

AND I'M ON THE ROAD AGAIN, roughly three years after the last time I did the cross-country drive. I seem to do them when I am in turmoil.

Disconnecting from my usual life patterns and driving for hours seems to help me recenter in some way. At least this time, I'm not in acute grief over the death of a partner, but I do figure I'm grieving in some rather odd ways, mainly connected to the ongoing saga of COVID that's defined all of our lives over the last 15 months.

COVID has led to lots of little deaths. Deaths of plans, deaths of certainties, deaths of possibilities. And then for me, there have been the very real deaths I've had to help people through—children grieving parents, parents grieving children, spouses grieving and adjusting to widowhood—as there are now 576,000 empty chairs at the American table and some of those are for my patients and their connections.

The vaccine has been a game-changer.

My patients, many cooped up for over a year, are able to venture out, some without being panicked, and families are able to gather together for the first time in a while. Even with that, the legacy of mental health conditions that has been left behind is enormous, and I'm only just beginning to unpack that particular box.

A large part of my day is spent working through grief, depression, and anxiety left in COVID's wake as that's now the major thing affecting my patients' health, far more than their blood pressure or their diabetes. I feel a bit inadequate to the task, but I usually muddle through somehow.

><>

I finished up my usual workday around 1:30 PM this afternoon, ran by the accountant to drop off my tax paperwork so I can get my refund, and then headed home to pack.

I like to travel and can usually pack pretty quickly and get supplies for anything from snowstorm to desert heat into a single suitcase. Just one of the things one learns growing up in Seattle when the weather can do anything over the course of a weekend.

Suitcases packed, trusty laptop in its bag, I kissed the kitties goodbye, threw things in the car, and headed out. I'm making this trip up as I go along. I have nearly a week to get to Seattle and a continent full of possible routes. We'll see where I end up.

I decided Northwest was as good a direction as any, so I took I-22 out of town past all the Walker County towns I know and love from VA house calls, and then on beyond into Mississippi. After Tupelo, which seems to have little reason for existing other than housing Elvis Presley's birthplace, (Will he be remembered in another few decades, after the Boomers are gone?), I drove into a glorious sunset straight out of Gone With the Wind for an hour or so as Mississippi gave way to Tennessee.

I figured Memphis was far enough for Day One. I stopped in the West suburbs, on the Arkansas side of the Mississippi, for the night.

With the crossing of the river, I guess I am officially in the West again. Can't say much about Memphis. The famous civic pyramid seems to have become a Bass Pro Shop, and it was too dark by the time I got to the bridge to see anything of Mud Island.

Tomorrow, I'll either head west toward Little Rock and Fort Smith or north toward St Louis. We'll see what I feel like after breakfast.

Twenty-three years ago, on our drive across the country from Sacramento to Birmingham to start our new life, Steve and I stopped for the night in Fort Smith. It was Halloween weekend and, while in the motel room, we turned on the TV and a local commercial blared for an Evangelical church's Harvest Festival party, an alternative to de-monic All-Hallow's Eve. Biblically correct costumes were encouraged.

Steve looked at me, rolled his eyes, and announced that he want-ed to stay an extra day so he could show up as Jezebel. He would have, too, if I had let him. But we had a van full of furniture to meet in Birmingham and could not afford the extra time.

My stops for gas and Dr. Pepper show that masks appear to be un-known here in the heartland. I'm trusting in my vaccinated status and wearing one when going indoors. I'm also keeping my hands washed and sanitized. And keeping a wide berth.

It's not over until it's over.

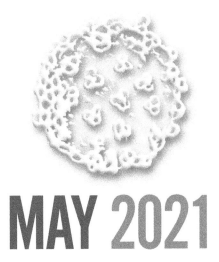

MAY 2021

See America First

SATURDAY | MAY 1, 2021

I HAVE A HEADACHE.

I don't usually get such things but I very definitely have a frontal headache tonight which started more or less when I got out of the car at tonight's Hampton Inn. I think it's just eye strain from driving all day. A couple of Tylenol and some rest should take care of it. But it is reminding me of how much I don't like not feeling well, especially when I'm not at home.

This last year or so of isolation not only kept me COVID-free, but it also kept me away from all of the other viruses and cruds I usually come into contact with. I've kind of forgotten what being under the weather feels like.

⚬⚬⚬

Today's drive was uneventful. West from Memphis across Arkansas (typical rural Americana), and then I decided to turn north and drive through the Ozarks. I had been through them once before with Steve on one of our trips when we were tracking down some 19th-century branch of his family tree, but I remember little about them.

What I found most interesting were the outcroppings of sedimentary rock sticking up from placid green hills, a gentle reminder that the central US was, for millennia, a vast inland sea. Things like this are reminders of how relatively unimportant anything going on today is in terms of geologic time. Six thousand years of recorded human history is the blink of an eye in the history of our planet.

The Ozarks these days bring two cultural touchstones to mind: Joan Hess' delightful Maggody murder mystery books and the recent Netflix series with Jason Bateman which suggests that rural Arkansas is full of feuding drug cartels. I did not see any drug lords but did pass what could have been the skeletal remains of Purtle's Esso station.

Descending from the Ozarks into Southern Missouri brought me to Branson where I managed to resist the siren call of theaters featuring Biblical spectaculars, acts from Hee-Haw, and half-forgotten comics. I also skipped the jeep tours through the cave, the indoor water parks, and the zipline adventures. I have no idea which of these may actually be in operation during these times of COVID, but the billboards live on.

Then on to Springfield, Joplin, and up a Missouri highway toward Kansas City that runs by a large Amish community. I passed four of their horse carriages and a number of barns with hex signs.

I'm stopping for the night on the outskirts of Kansas City and considering what tomorrow might bring. No matter how you slice it, it's likely to be the Great Plains.

I looked over COVID coverage this evening. Most of the articles are about the slow down in vaccination rates as the portion of the population seeking vaccine has been accommodated and the portion of the population avoiding vaccine remains constant. I don't know how to solve that one. I'm not certain that government mandates over our currently divided population are going to be helpful.

I think this may start solving itself through the marketplace. As COVID becomes more and more of a preventable disease, the health insurance industry will become less and less interested in paying for its costs in those who are eligible for vaccine but refuse. I suspect we'll start to see insurance companies requiring surcharges, much as they do with smokers, or having riders to their policies excluding coverage for COVID complications in those who could have been vaccinated. We shall see.

I saw a couple of carrion birds while driving through the Ozarks. They might have been buzzards or vultures or maybe even eagles. They didn't get close enough for me to tell. Vultures always remind me of my senior year in college. I had the same roommate through most of my undergraduate years at Stanford. The system that threw us together as freshmen did something right as we were quite compatible. During my sophomore year, we became good friends with a woman a few years older than us who had recently graduated but was still in the area working in theater, both on campus and off. It was the same year that Sondheim's Merrily We Roll Along crashed and burned on Broadway, and we always thought that the trio "Old Friends" was very much a song for us three. Our older friend did eventually get theater jobs away from campus and ended up working for the Oregon Shakespeare Festival in Ashland and was up there for the season. The problem was, the season ended in October and didn't begin again until February and without income, she couldn't pay rent during that off period.

My roommate and I, our senior year, had enough stage carpentry experience that we decided to build a loft for our dorm room. Stanford's dorms at that point dated mainly from the 40s and 50s and you more or less had a twelve-by-twelve cube to work with. Another dorm on campus, Toyon, had solved the lack of floor space problems for years with a loft system that was handed down from year to year and we thought we could replicate something like that in our dorm, Florence Moore Hall, or Flo Mo, on the other side of campus. We constructed quite the serviceable loft with two elevated beds at seven feet off the floor and a built-in carpet-covered couch/cot lower down.

Our dorm that year was a co-ed four-year dorm of three floors with about 70 kids and 3 resident assistants. I don't know what barrel the RAs were scraped out of that year, but we had three of the more clueless and unhelpful ones on campus (I don't remember any of their names). Because of this, the freshmen were kind of at sea, so my roommate and I more or less took them under our wing. Our room soon became the center of social life on our floor with late-night Trivial Pursuit and the freshmen feeling like they had seniors whom they could talk to.

We knew about our female friend's essential homelessness from November to February and hit upon a bright idea. She could come spend the time on campus, direct a musical revue, and stay in our dorm room. And so, she moved in, sleeping on the built-in couch. We got her an extra key from somewhere and she just became part of dorm life. Most of the girls, who saw her in the bathroom in the morning, thought she was someone who lived at the other end of the hall whom they hadn't gotten to know yet, and the clueless RAs, so wrapped up in themselves, never noticed that the population of the dorm increased by one for three months. (She did go home to her parents over the Christmas break).

When it was time for her to go back to Ashland, she gave me a stuffed vulture. She says that the first thing she would see in the morning was me peering over the edge of my loft bed, looking as to where I could jump down without landing on her. I still have it. Going to find a bad movie and go blah for the next few hours.

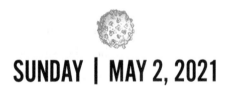

SUNDAY | MAY 2, 2021

THE HEADACHE WENT AWAY but I still wasn't feeling great this morning when I headed back down the road.

After a few hours, it became clear that my original plan to haul myself all the way to Denver was not the best of ideas as it would require more driving hours than might be good for me. I'd rather not fall asleep at the wheel and run off the road if I can avoid it. So I ticked off the Kansas towns as they went by—Topeka, Junction City, Salina.

Looking ahead on I-70, it became clear that by the time I hit the high plains of Western Kansas and Eastern Colorado, there would be a paucity of population centers and Hampton Inns, so I turned right at Salina, headed up through Kansas and Nebraska farmland, and stopped early in Grand Island, Nebraska for a nap before dinner and family Zoom night conversation thereafter.

Not much to say about the Prairie. It goes on forever and is very flat. Most of the fields visible from the highway are beige, spring stubble endowing it with the sepia tone of the Kansas sequences from *The Wizard of Oz*. I can't say much about Grand Island either, other than it's the home of the Nebraska State Fair and one of the heartland towns that had a terrible COVID outbreak earlier in the pandemic.

I'm keeping away from the natives, snuggled up here in my hotel room as it begins to rain, bolts of lightning vying with the green and red of the Applebee's sign that dominates the view from my hotel room window for the attention of my visual cortex.

>━●

I don't think I've got any good stories about driving across the Great Plains.

Tommy and I never did it together. Steve and I did it more times than I care to count. Among other things, Steve was a genealogist who kept himself busy tracing all of the Spivey descendants from the three Spivey brothers who originally immigrated to the Ashville, NC area in the 1760s.

We would pack up the truck and head out for a couple of weeks in the courthouses of the Midwest and Appalachia looking for clues. He did the driving, and I read to him. He was partial to long works of historical fiction.

In later years, when I had routine work in DC, he would come with me. We would rent a car and head south, removing the need to cross the empty quarter of the continent. This was all before GPS and smartphones, and there would be any number of fights over the large road Atlas as we tried to figure out the best way to get to some small county seat in Arkansas or Tennessee or Kentucky.

During one of these trips, late in the year, we were driving along I-65 through Kentucky when it began to snow. Steve, having been raised a Southern California boy, had never actually seen snowfall before. We pulled over at the next rest stop so he could caper about, catch snowflakes with his tongue, and enjoy all of those usual childhood rites of passage that had been denied him until his forties.

Steve always had an idiosyncratic approach to life. We used to travel a lot with the gay travel group Atlantis Events and, in January of 1999, shortly after we had moved to Birmingham, we were booked on one of their very first Caribbean cruises. This was before Steve became ill, so he was in fine form, making sure he was noticed by the other guests and staff alike. Steve was always happiest when he was the center of attention. He didn't much care if it was positive or negative. The special guest entertainer on the cruise was Chaka Khan and one evening, she did her set. Later that night, there was a white party up on the deck. For those not of the gay male dance party persuasion, a white party is one in which the attendees are expected to wear white outfits or costumes; it usually ends up as a lot of guys in their underwear. It was a lovely warm night on the Caribbean Sea so most of the men weren't wearing a whole lot. Steve decided to attend wearing a white sailor midi blouse top, a white sailor hat, and a white jock strap. The top was long enough to cover most of his rump, not that that crowd cared, and he and I were dancing under the stars. Chaka came out on deck and sat at a table at the side of the dance floor to watch the dancing and Steve spotted her. He immediately took off his jock strap, tossed it in her direction, and then proceeded to flash her. Her response was uproarious laughter and something along the lines of "Honey, a girl likes it when you leave something to the imagination". He laughed back and she invited us to sit down with her. Steve and she were roughly the same age, knew some of the same people in LA, and soon were having a high old time together, even if he wasn't wearing any pants. He always adored African-American women and they him. Once we moved to Birmingham, he would say the most outrageous things to African-American women we would encounter and they would all laugh, and then fix him with an amused, but steely gaze and say, "You're so bad," to which his standard response was, "I didn't know any better," and they would all laugh again.

For those of you who were wondering, yes, I had my pants on, thank you very much. If I recall correctly, I was wearing white jeans and some sort of sheer white top. Yes, there are photos. No, I'm not publishing them. To this day, it remains the only time I've had cock-tails with a celebrity while my husband was naked from the waist down.

More Great Plains tomorrow and then into the Rockies.

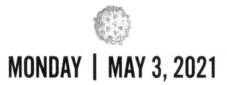

MONDAY | MAY 3, 2021

DON'T KNOW WHAT WAS WRONG WITH ME YESTERDAY.
But ending my driving early, going to bed, and sleeping for
ten hours was the right decision. I felt pretty much back to normal
today and had no difficulty with a long drive of over 600 miles.

My initial thought was to cut back down to Denver and cross
through the Rockies on I-70. Then I checked the weather report
which announced a significant winter storm in central Colorado with
up to a foot of snow. I decided that might not be the best of ideas, so I
stayed on I-80 through Nebraska and into Wyoming.

It started to snow as I passed through Cheyenne and continued
to do so through the mountains surrounding Laramie. It wasn't more
than a dusting. It didn't cause too many problems—other than issues
with visibility like the entire world being reduced to shades of gray
and white between snow, clouds, and mountains. It was all over, by
the time I hit the Continental Divide. I coasted on into the exciting
town of Rock Springs, Wyoming without incident.

I can't say much about today's drive. Western Nebraska is flat. The
highway seems to continuously cross various branches of the Platte
River (so named after the French word for "flat"). It's a steady incline in
elevation over the miles, barely noticeable. Then you're in the mountains of Wyoming, heading over passes at 8,500 feet.

On the other side of the mountains come miles and miles of high
plains scrubland full of sagebrush and sweeping skies, needing only
Clint Eastwood to complete the picture. I have two days of driving left
to Seattle. I'm not sure of my route yet. I'll check out weather maps
tonight before making a final decision.

The news from Covidland today was not good.

CDC experts are despairing of the US population achieving anything like herd immunity due to the political unpopularity of vaccines in certain quarters. What does this mean? It means COVID is likely to be with us for years, decades, permanently.

I don't think we need to panic about this as individuals.

Those with a belief in science and a couple of hundred years of epidemiological understanding will be OK. Among those who don't, or who belong to less privileged communities that are more difficult to reach with vaccine and the like, the disease will continue to spread and pop up in epidemic fashion. We'll continue to see serious illness and death, but not in the numbers of the last year. It didn't have to be this way, but that's the political reality we have to live—and die—with.

I'm starting to get a little worried about the next couple of election cycles. The speed with which the Republican party is whitewashing the Capitol Insurrection and various other criminal enterprises, combined with a complacency among the Democrats now that vaccines are distributed, makes me think that maintaining congressional majorities is going to be difficult.

If there is a shift in power at the midterms, all of the social trends that have led to an anti-science/anti-knowledge/anti-Enlightenment approach to governance will come roaring back emboldened. Who knows what sort of national problem they will intersect with to cause some other sort of disaster? (Rant over.)

Time for some bad TV and sleep.

TUESDAY | MAY 4, 2021

'M DEFINITELY BACK IN THE WEST and heading into my old stomping grounds.

Today's drive wasn't difficult. I started in Southwest Wyoming, along Interstate 80 over the border to Utah, threaded through the various canyons and mountain ranges outside of Ogden, then up into the Snake River country of Idaho. Finally, I reached the flat valley of the Boise River and the city of Boise itself.

Thirty-five years ago, I spent a summer in Boise with a couple of wild women doing my OB/GYN clerkship. We lived together on the upper floor of an old house containing a local OB/GYN practice, We spent our time catching babies at St Luke's hospital and observing gynecological surgery at St. Al's across town.

The house is still standing. The practice is not. It dissolved not too long after our summer there. We medical students had ferreted out an inappropriate relationship between one of the partners and the office manager. We weren't going to say anything but we did make bets about how long that was going to go on before it caused an explosion.

I don't remember too much about downtown Boise from that summer. It was hot. The downtown area was tired and old, stuck in a decaying 1950s-60s. By contrast, the Boise of today appears to be in growth mode, like a lot of older cities. Much of downtown has been redone with new restaurants, bars, hotels, and businesses, and the millennials are flocking to new housing units in old buildings. A block away from my hotel is The Basque Block, a collection of Basque restaurants, a Basque grocery, the Basque cultural center, and some upscale watering holes. I had a very nice meal under a large Basque flag.

As I was sitting there looking at the millennials having their dinner and drinks, I couldn't help but wonder if I delivered any of them. All those babies are turning 35 this summer and are likely parents themselves.

I also wondered what I might say to 24-year-old Andy if I were to meet him coming down the street. If he would even begin to believe some of the twists and turns that life was going to start throwing his way shortly after that summer. I doubt I would have believed any of it. At 24, I was just trying to get through medical school with my sanity intact and wasn't really thinking about much else.

Highlights of that summer were inner tubing down the Boise River and a side trip to Yellowstone and the Grand Tetons. The actual OB/GYN work was not a highlight, although I did like playing with the newborns. I just wish I hadn't had to send some of them home with their parents who were obviously ill-equipped for the rigors of child-rearing.

><@>

I often wonder if whether Steve and I or Tommy and I would have been capable of child-rearing ourselves. They both loved kids and loved to play, each in their own way. The timing was always wrong for us to work seriously towards children of our own, so we had to play in our own ways.

Steve and I had always enjoyed fun-in-the-sun vacations and went on a lot of them over the years. A lot of them run together in my mind but they were mainly to Hawaii and Mexico.

When Tommy and I got together, I assumed we would have a similar pattern. I hadn't counted on Tommy's Irish coloring and skin which did not mix well with tropical sun. Just walking across the pool area, even with SPF 1000 sunblock was enough to turn him bright pink, and he usually had to hide out in the shade somewhere.

He didn't have great skin to begin with and sunburn just made everything worse. We did go on a few, but they were far less common than I had been used to.

One of Tommy and my few tropical vacations was in early 2005. We started to get involved in the world of Birmingham theater together less than a year previously and we were still in our pre-theatrical patterns. I had just spent a couple of years getting the new geriatric clinic at UAB up and running and Tommy was the chief nursing officer at an outfit called Birmingham Health Care, a collection of federally qualified health centers providing care to low-income individuals.

I booked us on an Atlantis Cruise together. Atlantis is an outfit that specializes in group vacations for gay men. Steve and I had been regulars with them, even before they did cruises, and Tommy and I had also been on a couple of trips. Dates had been submitted to employers, everything was cleared through our various bureaucracies, and we were to fly out Saturday to catch the boat in Miami. On the Friday, just before, Tommy's boss called him into his office, told him that a major grant was due right after we were due to return, and he expected it finished and on his desk. Tommy, with his incredible work ethic, simply took the grant with us. We spent the cruise in the cabin working on his grant. I was livid.

When we got back, I told Tommy in no uncertain terms that good people did not do things like that to their employees, and it was time for him to leave that job. He thought about it for a while, and ultimately did decide to go about six months later. It was the first step on the road that took him back to school at the University of Montevallo and his new career(s).

Years later we figured out what was really going on. Tommy, in addition to being chief nursing officer, was also ethics/compliance officer for the organization. Unbeknownst to him, his boss and the senior staff had cooked up a number of schemes to enrich themselves through various unethical and illegal means off of federal contracts and they knew Tommy would never stand for it so he had to be made miserable enough to quit.

He had the last laugh. The federal government eventually caught on to their hanky-panky, the organization collapsed and most of the senior staff has either gone to jail or spent most of their money on lawyers to keep them out. We read the newspaper reports of the spectacular implosion and various criminal proceedings with relish and appropriate schadenfreude. One more day of driving and I should be in Seattle in time for dinner.

SATURDAY | MAY 8, 2021

TIME TO CHECK IN.

I can tell that I'm pretty unplugged from life because I keep falling asleep if I sit still for more than about five minutes.

Nothing terribly exciting has happened the last few days. I've had family time, a meeting with my editor, some time with friends, and a lot of napping. It may not be the most action-packed of weeks, but I think it's what I've needed.

I have two more days here. I depart on Tuesday for the trek back across the country. I've figured out the first two-thirds of that based on time, distances, and weather. I'm going to leave the last third up to happenstance when I get there.

⤜⊶

Seattle is home and also not.

My relationship with the city is very much of the You-Can't-Go Home-Again variety. The Seattle I grew up in during the 1960s and

1970s no longer truly exists. It pokes through from time to time like a pentimento, but newer trends and sights and people have long since transformed the small city of my childhood into something else.

The Seattle of my past was a city of self-sufficient neighborhoods, each a village of friends and neighbors who knew and supported each other. Each one had its own small commercial district where the majority of business was done. A trip to the mall or downtown was a significant event. The geography of the town—you could only go so far before running into a lake or a ravine —kept the various regions insular and small-town feeling.

Downtown, when I was a child, was dominated by the Seattle Center and the Space Needle, the old World's Fair grounds at one end, Pioneer Square and Smith Tower at the other. There wasn't all that much in between—a few high rises dating back to the 20s and a lot of undistinguished post-war stuff filling in the rest. The Pike Place Market was there, but had not yet become a fish-flinging tourist mecca, and there was a great deal of discussion about tearing it down as it had become rickety and in poor repair over the years.

Things started to change in the early 70s.

I can remember pretty much when all of the modern skyscrapers went up, starting with what was the SeaFirst Bank tower (now Safeco Plaza), joined by box after box of chromium steel and tinted windows going up routinely over the next couple of decades until they started to run out of room. Now, as the tech giants expand, more and more buildings are going up South of Lake Union, and whole sections of town are unrecognizable.

The huge growth in tech has led to a huge influx of people. The city itself has about 50% more people than the city of my youth. The metro area is nearly twice as populous. As the city is hemmed in by water, it has minimal land area for expansion. This has led to increased density, increased real estate prices, and increased pressure on public goods and services.

The neighborhoods of middle-class homes are being bulldozed for multi-family dwellings, and workingmen's bungalows are being replaced by large modern homes, often in a horrifically unattractive boxy style that makes them look like an ugly dentist's office of the 1970s. The rapid increase in rents has pushed some of the poor out of housing entirely. Many of the parks and public green spaces are sprouting tent colonies.

Perhaps one of the things that keeps me in Birmingham is that the feel of the city is similar to what Seattle once was.

When I go out in Birmingham in my part of the city, I am apt to run into friends and acquaintances (at least in non-COVID times). There's a feeling of community among those of us professionals of a more liberal persuasion who choose to live in the city itself rather than in the suburbs. It's an urban environment, but small enough to be manageable and, for someone like me, to feel connected to the life and health of the city as a whole, so I feel I can support it and that can support me. I'm not sure that Seattle could do that for me these days.

Seattle, as ground zero for COVID in the long-ago days of March 2020, continues to take things relatively seriously. Most citizens are wearing masks indoors without complaint. Outdoor dining is popular, and it's warm enough now for it to be comfortable, so I've been taking advantage of that. The majority of the citizenry is in the process of receiving their vaccinations. I haven't felt unsafe at all during this visit.

Vaccination rates, in general, are starting to fall off significantly as those with interest and who have been pursuing them have achieved their goals. Roughly 1/3 of the US population is now totally vaccinated. We'll hit about 1/2 over the next month as all the vaccinations in process are completed.

I figure we'll end up somewhere around 60%. Not enough for

herd immunity by a long shot.

What should we do as a society to increase that number? I am uncertain. There are significant ethical and other issues at play with any potential plan. I'm going to cogitate on this a bit and maybe I'll get back to it in another musing.

In the meantime, mask up indoors with others, wash your hands, and keep your distance.

TUESDAY | MAY 11, 2021

HAPPY BIRTHDAY TO ME.

One more year until another milestone and another decade. I tend to alternate between good and bad decades with the even ones being good ones. Hopefully, my 60s will be kind to me when they get here. God knows I'm becoming far older than I ever intended to be, but that's the way of the world.

We all age at exactly the same chronological rate, but the physiological aspects vary a bit depending on genetics, environment, and life choices. Somewhere close to 600 people have messaged, texted, Facebooked, called, or otherwise let me know they were thinking of me today. I am reading and responding to everyone, but it may be a few days before I get to all of them.

Scrolling through Facebook well-wishes is always interesting. As each familiar name goes by, it brings up images of the time in my life when that person entered it. Childhood playmates, school friends, colleagues, people in the opera and theater worlds, vacation buddies— each important and each a reminder of how many people we touch as we go through life. Sources tell me I even got a shout-out on

Birmingham Mountain Radio this morning. That's a new one.

The last few days in Seattle were uneventful. I got some writing done, did my usual geriatric Q-and-A for my father's senior community residents (only this time, it had to be done via video rather than in person due to COVID precautions), and had some time with old friends.

The immediate family gathered for my birthday dinner last night. Everyone was well and made merry over a salmon dinner. This morning, I had breakfast with my father. I admonished him again not to leave his building without his stick for improved balance, received his birthday blessings, and headed out on the return journey.

Rather than head directly east, I first went north and had coffee and a long chat with my college roommate, who has relocated from Alaska to Bellingham. That put me in position to cross the Cascades via the North Cascades Highway and Washington Pass, a road I had not taken for decades.

The pass doesn't open until late in the season due to the snow. It had only been clear for about a week, so there was little traffic. There was a good foot of snow on the ground but none on the pavement. The weather was spectacular, allowing for amazing views of Liberty Bell mountain and surrounding peaks. My favorite mountain pass remains Logan Pass in Glacier National Park, but this one is a close second and is far less known.

From the mountains, I headed down the Methow Valley and then over various back roads of Eastern Washington. I crossed the Columbia River at Chief Joseph Dam, and an hour later passed Grand Coulee Dam in its canyon, before heading on to Spokane for the night. It has been many decades since I was last on most of these roads, some of them not since childhood. Various sites and place names brought up memories of family vacation road trips of the 1970s.

Grand Coulee Dam always makes me think of my father, who worships at the altar of Woody Guthrie and Pete Seeger, piloting first a station wagon, and later a van, full of family and camping equipment, singing Roll On, Columbia, Roll On with its verses celebrating various Washington state sites. Or passing the sign to Ritzville and remembering my sister at roughly age six, being vastly disappointed to find that the town was not made of crackers.

Tomorrow is more mountain driving through the Rockies. The weather promises to be fair, so it should be uneventful as long as I remember to keep myself well-caffeinated.

WEDNESDAY | MAY 12, 2021

TODAY WAS A STRAIGHT 540-MILE SHOT ON I-90.

Not so straight, actually, as it ran primarily through mountain country. Lots of ups, downs, S-curves, slow trucks, views of lakes, mountain peaks, and rushing rivers that only needed a young Brad Pitt in hip waders to be complete.

The weather is holding. There is no gas shortage in this part of the country. Hampton Inns are pretty much the same everywhere you go.

From Spokane the road curves along Lake Coeur D'Alene in Idaho while crossing the panhandle and then climbs up into the mountain country of Western Montana. The passes were all clear of snow, even at the 6500-foot level of the Continental Divide outside of Butte. All of the clusters of mountains have range names, but they are part of the same cordillera that contains the Rockies, so I have always thought of them as the northern Rockies.

Once up in the high plateau, it's mainly the broad river valleys of the Missouri headwaters and the Yellowstone. I bypassed the park on its northern border after going through Missoula and Bozeman, eventually arriving at Billings which was far enough to go in one drive.

><>

Many years ago, I spent a month or so in Western Montana, north of Kalispell, in the town of Whitefish, long before it became a trendy Western mecca for the well-heeled. I was there to do my rotation in Family Practice, attached to a group of physicians who were the major providers in town and first-call to the emergency department at their tiny rural hospital. I was responsible for the after-hours emergency department calls to do a preliminary evaluation and warrant whether a "real" doctor needed to be woken up.

Drunk tourist with a bellyache? I could handle that. Gored by a bull? As the wound was in the belly, that had to be loaded up in an ambulance and taken to Kalispell for surgical evaluation. Fell off a horse on a trail ride and sustained a Colle's wrist fracture? Apply splint and help them arrange for orthopedic follow-up when they get back home to Minnesota. It was one of the experiences that taught me how to think well on my feet, and one which kept me from being afraid of rural medicine, or of delivering care without a tertiary care university hospital hovering behind me.

><>

Whitefish is just outside of Glacier National Park. I was in the park on day hikes every day off. I got one long weekend during my time there and used that to head up to Banff/Jasper where I had not been since I was a tot of four—a trip long remembered in family lore: the engine fell out of the car in the middle of the Banff Jasper highway, leading to a number of complications.

I want to go back to Glacier/Banff/Jasper/Waterton Lakes as a mature adult and see them all again. Perhaps after I retire, I'll take a leisurely trip out to Seattle and spend some time going all the way up the Rockies from Denver, taking in the Tetons, Yellowstone, and the others mentioned above.

Then again, I might skip Waterton Lakes. The last time I was there, around age 12, a deer came up to me in the campground. When I had nothing to feed it, it reared up on its hind legs and planted both its forehooves in the middle of my chest, knocking me over, before stalking off in search of another campsite where people might be freer with the treats.

My encounters with deer and elk this trip have been less dramatic. I've seen them only in passing from the car. No bear this trip, either. I can do without seeing a grizzly in the wild, but I don't mind the occasional black bear encounter. I've had a number of those over the years. The bear is usually not at all interested and ambles off in another direction. The only one that was at all unusual was when I was four on the same Banff trip when the car fell apart.

My mother was reading to me in the tent when our dog, Duffy, a West Highland White terrier who was tied up outside, began to bark. This was unusual, so my mother stuck her head out of the tent and discovered a large black bear pawing at things in the next campsite. She scooped me up and took off down the road where we took refuge at the ranger station.

My father, when he came back from dealing with car trouble, was glad we were OK (the bear having been chased off by the rangers), but was upset at my mother for having not grabbed up the dog at the same time she grabbed me. The dog was fine. The bear wasn't the least bit interested in yapping terriers.

Down from the mountains and onto the plains tomorrow.

THURSDAY | MAY 13, 2021

REALIZED AS I STUDIED THE MAP LAST NIGHT that I had two choices for today.

I could cut things a little short and spend the night in Rapid City, South Dakota, on the western border of the state, or I could power through and drive nearly 700 miles and spend the night in Sioux Falls on the eastern border of the state.

There is nothing between them other than Wall Drug, and I had no interest in bunking there for the night. I decided, as the weather was not the best and I was dodging rain showers all day, that it would be wise to choose the former course and end early.

From Billings, the road veers southeast and passes the Little Big Horn battlefield, site of Custer's famed defeat. As I was in no hurry, I stopped for a while. I had been here once before several decades ago. It hasn't changed much: rolling hills above the Little Big Horn river dotted with white marble markers where the 7th Cavalry fell.

Fortunately, we are starting to wake up to the fact that the "taming of the West" is a complex story.

It's probably best not to celebrate genocidal wars without acknowledging the other side, so there are now exhibits celebrating the Lakota and Oglala Sioux, Cheyenne, Arapahoe, and other indigenous people involved in a battle to preserve their way of life—and brown marble markers placed where their warriors died.

I also noted that the Lewis and Clark trail historical markers have been redesigned to include Sacagawea and her baby which is only fitting. The road then crosses into the high mountain plains of northeast Wyoming for a few hundred miles, entering South Dakota in the Black Hills, just north of Deadwood.

By this time, it was raining so my thoughts of detouring to Deadwood and Mount Rushmore fell by the wayside. Heading up into the mountains in a rainstorm seemed like a bad idea. Besides, I'd already been there on a previous visit to the region. So I had an early dinner in Rapid City and checked into the Hampton Inn where I found I had been upgraded to what I take is their honeymoon suite from the large jacuzzi tub in the living room. After three days of driving, a nice hot bath with jets seemed like a swell idea, so I filled it up and soaked for a bit.

›—◁

I turned on the news in time to catch the CDC's announcement that masks would no longer be required indoors for the fully vaccinated in uncrowded situations. The number of vaccinated adults has continued to increase, especially in urban areas. A dozen states are above 2/3 of their population vaccinated.

In Seattle, the neighborhoods where my family live are over 80% vaccinated. This is leading to a precipitous fall in deaths, if not total cases, the disease having been pushed into a younger cohort less likely to be vaccinated but also less likely to die.

I hadn't checked the nationwide statistics for a while so I looked them up. About 33 million US cases (roughly 10% of the population) and about 584,000 deaths to date.

I'm starting to wonder if this means the end of *The Accidental Plague Diaries*? They've occupied a lot of the last 14 months of my life. Part of me would hope so, but I don't think this story is over yet by a long shot. Our current political climate is going to ensure that.

Despite the incredible biomedical effort that the development and administration of a vaccine in just over a year represents, we still have a major political party dancing around full of delusions regarding the operation of science, medicine, and public health. The more time goes by, the more delusional it appears to become. At the moment, it's trying to gaslight the entire world into believing that what occurred on January 6th was not what was recorded and played out in real time in front of all of our horrified eyes.

I have to get back into my usual groove and off the road to start thinking about all this a bit more. Then I'll be able to give a better assessment about what I think of the COVID-19 endgame and what is likely to come next.

FRIDAY | MAY 14, 2021

NOTHER UNEXCITING DRIVE across the Great Plains today. From Rapid City, the road descends out of the Black Hills onto the plain and then runs more or less in a straight line for hundreds of miles. It's flat, farm country, pretty much featureless. An hour or so to the east of the hill country is the nothing town of Wall, South Dakota, home to Wall Drug, a small business possessed of an infinite capacity for self-promotion with essentially no competition in a several-hundred-mile radius.

I passed the billboards. I did not stop as I visited the establishment on my last trip across I-90 and generally don't feel a need to return to tourist traps of no consequence.

More and more flatlands, with the Badlands on the horizon to the south, and the occasional sign pointing to DeSmet (the little town on the prairie where Laura Ingalls Wilder spent her girlhood) or the Corn Palace. I stopped for lunch at that exit and then drove past. It's a Shriners' auditorium covered with corn husks.

At Sioux Falls, right turn from I-90 to I-29, south for a few hundred miles out of South Dakota, across the Missouri River (again), and into Iowa at Sioux City. More flatlands and then there are the few towers of Omaha rising up looking like a less colorful Emerald City.

My Hampton Inn of the evening turned out to be right across the river in Council Bluffs, part of a complex of hotels on the water, revolving around a Riverboat casino that, while technically on the water, has obviously never sailed anywhere. The CDC may be loosening restrictions, but jostling around middle America feeding one-arm bandits did not appeal, so I took a walk around the outside before retiring for the evening.

><>

I'm still trying to digest the change in CDC guidance regarding indoor masking that came down yesterday and how I should apply it in my life. There are a few salient points.

The CDC did not say that it is safe for people to gather indoors unmasked. It said it was safe for *fully vaccinated* people to gather indoors unmasked and that most normal activities are safe for them. They are not safe for unvaccinated people.

What does this mean in practical terms? I think if you are gathering privately with family or friends and everyone is vaccinated, there's nothing to worry about. Larger public gatherings are still problematic as not everyone who wishes a vaccine has been able to obtain one. And there remains a significant subset of the population refusing vaccination, largely for political reasons.

There's no way to tell who has been vaccinated and who has not other than self-report. There's been discussion of vaccine passports on smartphones, but this will leave out the significant population of folks who can't use a smartphone and folks who can't afford such devices. So I have reservations about such a system. And having uniformed people at the entrance of a place of public gathering demanding *"Papieren bitte!"* brings up images of totalitarianism we just don't need.

I've opined before that the liability insurance industry is likely to begin writing the rules going forward as they will not want to indemnify businesses depending on people coming together if the business does not have a plan to prevent the spread of pandemic disease in place.

Variants of various stripes are spreading. They will all eventually reach the US and will pass into the unvaccinated population and be spread. We live in such an interconnected world that pandemic disease is a global problem, not a national problem. We've been so preoccupied with our issues here and how the previous administration dropped the ball, that we've been paying very little attention to what's been going on elsewhere in the world.

From what we know so far, the vaccines are protecting against spread and serious disease from variants. The mRNA technology behind the Pfizer and Moderna vaccines is such that tweaks can be made quickly. We're unlikely to be caught in a situation as we were last winter but anything is possible. We may need to keep getting COVID boosters going forward. I'd rather have a booster than a ventilator any day.

There were a number of reports today about the spread of COVID in the fully vaccinated New York Yankees organization. People have tested positive. One person was mildly symptomatic but most were asymptomatic. It doesn't look like anyone is getting seriously ill.

That's the thing to remember here. The vaccines aren't perfect in regard to protection against infection. What's important is that they offer a very high level of protection against serious disease requiring hospitalization. If we test widely, we're going to find a lot of asymptomatic infections; the virus isn't going away. But as long as people aren't getting seriously ill, I wouldn't worry a lot about these reports.

It's going to be problematic, however, if the disease gets into organizations catering to those refusing vaccine for political reasons. We're going to continue to see spread and serious illness and death in these situations. I don't know what we can do about it.

Private entities can mandate vaccine as a condition of employment or entry, but we've so weakened the ability of government to do this, at the behest of concerned parents of the anti-vaxxer movement over the last few decades, that it will be difficult to get government involved in any way other than an advisory role.

Brunch with a friend tomorrow! Then further southward.

SATURDAY | MAY 15, 2021

TONIGHT IS MY LAST NIGHT ON THE ROAD.

I'll make the drive home tomorrow. The day after I will plug back into my usual life and patterns. These two weeks of unplugging have been good for me, but it's time to get back to those who depend on me in one way or another at work and with life in general.

I'll be in normal patterns through the summer and, in September, I'll get to break away again assuming that COVID doesn't mutate in such a way as to shut travel back down. Anything is possible with this disease. We're fooling ourselves if we think the last chapters of the saga have been written. I'm sure there is more to come; I just don't yet know what form it is likely to take.

Today started with a Drag Brunch in Council Bluffs, Iowa. (Now there's a sentence I never thought I'd write.) A friend whom I have known and corresponded with since the early days of Epinions and my Mrs. Norman Maine film review columns, but whom I had never actually met, lives in the area. I suggested we get together for brunch.

Her researches turned up a decent place in downtown Council Bluffs and, as luck would have it, today was their once-a-month Saturday brunch with drag queen entertainment. How could we not?

She had a breakfast sandwich; I had French toast. We caught up and were entertained by beefy country boys in bodysuits, wigs that Tommy would want to restyle, and excessive pancake, busy lip-synching to disco hits popular before they were born. It was lovely. Unfortunately, I could not order the drinks served in small fish bowls as I had a 600-mile drive in front of me.

After departing Council Bluffs, I headed south along the Missouri River, eventually ending up on the opposite end of Kansas City from the end I hit on my outbound trip. There I turned east, crossed Missouri to St. Louis, became very confused by the interchanges leading from I-70 to I-64, and had to get off the highway downtown near the Gateway Arch in order to figure it back out. Eventually, I found the right road out of town.

Then across Southern Illinois, and into the Southern tip of Indiana, stopping tonight in Evansville. None of the scenery was terribly exciting —typical rolling hills, some woodlands, and a lot of pastureland. Also an inordinate number of dead deer on the roadside. Fortunately, I did not hit any.

><>

I picked Evansville deliberately.

In this town, 73 years ago, Jon Steven Spivey made his entrance into the world. His father was from Crawfordsville, his mother from Russellville, both in Northern Indiana. Steve was a little hazy about how the family had ended up in the southern part of the state.

There was some story about his father needing to make a geographic relocation to stay a step ahead of some unspecified trouble.

He never said for certain, but I believe it was alcohol-related. Alcohol issues tended to follow the Spivey men. Steve was 30 years sober when he died.

When Steve was four, the family made another major geographic relocation to suburban LA (Sun Valley in the San Fernando Valley, just a bit north of Studio City). That was where he grew up. To my knowledge, Steve never returned to Evansville and the two of us never passed through on any of our Midwest/Appalachian trips when he was doing his genealogical research, so I thought I would take this chance to at least see what it looks like. I wasn't impressed.

My audiobook for the last few days has been Isabelle Wilkerson's Caste which has got me thinking about a whole lot of issues, but I'm going to need to think about them for a few days before even thinking about writing about them. Until then, bad television, a good night's sleep, and home tomorrow before dinner time.

TUESDAY | MAY 18, 2021

RETURNING BACK TO WORK after being away for a few weeks is always painful.

I have piles of papers requiring signatures, multiple mailboxes, both regular and e-, to empty and sort, and there's always a subtle sense of something vital that got missed along the way. You know it's going to reappear later and with innumerable complications, usually at an inopportune time.

I've had a full day at the UAB half of my job and another full day at the VA half. Things aren't yet fully caught up, but there's a plan in place to get everything back where it belongs by the end of the week.

Many of my patients and their families seem to think that only I can help with the latest issue. I trust my teams and colleagues implicitly and have them well trained. They do just fine in my absence, even if they are met by grumbling at times that it's not me. I wonder what they're all going to do in a few years when I announce my retirement? I'm not exactly sure when that will be. Sometime between 2024 and 2029 I expect. I'm keeping my options open.

><>

I will be bowing out in time to not have to deal with the enormous problems that "peak age" are going to bring to the health system. This happens between 2030 and 2035. It's the time when the entire Baby Boom will be over the age of 65 and eligible for Medicare, but will not yet have entered their major die-off. That will start in full force around 2032 and accelerate through the early 2040s, ending around 2050 or so.

The Baby Boom generation will lose its grip on social power in the late 2030s and will basically be irrelevant around 2050. At that time, the oldest boomers will be 104 (Cher will be doing another farewell tour.); the youngest will be 86.

In 2060, the boomers will be what World War II veterans are today: a few still around to be celebrated, but the vast majority gone. They will continue to linger on until the very last one dies in roughly 2080 when one of the youngest boomers, almost certainly female, born in 1963 or 1964, will die at the age of 116 or so.

The book I was writing, pre-COVID, was about this phenomenon and my predictions regarding the impact of the Boom on the healthcare system over the next decade, as the irresistible force of an aging generation with an expectation of eternal youth meets the immovable object of biological aging and the structure of the healthcare system. Maybe I'll return to it. COVID sidetracked it into *The Accidental Plague Diaries*.

I'm still not sure what to make of the most recent CDC guidance regarding vaccination and masking. I understand that they're trying to use "Vaccination = Ditch the Mask" as a selling point to get those on the fence in for their jabs, but it does seem as if it creates a sort of nationwide honor system regarding vaccination status. There's no way to tell if the nice person smiling at you is fully vaccinated or a rabid anti-masker who believes in vaccine microchips and other such nonsense and is a potential source of contagion.

If the last few years have taught me anything, it's that I need to be wary of the American population as a whole. They have shown themselves not to be the most trustworthy, and it strikes me that a significant part of the population has dumped the Golden Rule and the other teachings of religion in favor of the collected philosophies of Ayn Rand and Roy Cohn.

We'll all find out if the current optimism regarding COVID is correct over the next month or so. The numbers are way down, the fourth wave that seemed to be developing in mid-Spring having sputtered out. Whether this is due to increasing vaccination rates or other phenomena is unclear.

The change in behavior over the last week or so with fewer restrictions will be reflected in infection rates around Memorial Day. If we've got it wrong, death rates will start going up again in mid-June.

I certainly hope we have it right, but I'm still being cautious. I put my mask on when I go indoors with people whose vaccination status I don't know. The issues of the unvaccinated and inequality in vaccine distribution pretty much all come down to "No one is alone."

We live in a complex interdependent world where the health of any of us depends on the health of each of us. Any group left behind or left out when it comes to pandemic illness can serve as the breeding ground for the next contagion.

We are lucky that this one is not more fatal than it has been. If the next thing that comes around has the mortality rate of Ebola, we'd be looking at wholesale societal collapse. And I'm not sure that Western societies, with their tilt away from public good to private gain, will be able to do better in the future with the next inevitable viral illness that comes along.

Have we learned lessons as a society that will stick with us? It's hard to say. The American attention span isn't all that long, and there are political and economic forces at work trying to downplay a lot of the bad that's been going on in society.

This isn't just limited to health issues. I read comments today from a sitting member of congress, photographed blockading the doors of the House chambers with furniture on the day of the insurrection, describing these events as nothing more than a bunch of tourists.

This makes me wonder what his family vacations were like. Did they storm Old Faithful waving flags and armed with assault rifles last summer? Perhaps they broke through the emergency doors of It's a Small World to make sure they got into the front of the boat.

There's an agenda at work here that I don't completely understand, but I'm trying to get a better sense of how it crosses with health policy. I'll let someone with more experience analyze the political trends.

SATURDAY | MAY 22, 2021

I'M BACK IN MY USUAL GROOVE.

I can tell because I fell asleep three times this afternoon while attempting to finish up my progress notes from this past week. I still have quite a number to go but have finished the batch that will be delinquent if they aren't done this weekend.

I write about 1500 of them a year. That's about 50,000 over the course of my career to date.

They have morphed from handwritten documents, to dictated notes transcribed by a specialist, to computer-assisted notes where the computer kept track of things like the med list but where I still dictated the meat of the note, to now full electronic health records, replete with little point-and-click boxes and various free text fields in which I have to type things, most dictated by payment systems, and not by clinical care.

I'm not sure if that's progress or not. My first job in high school was as a keypunch operator working with Hollerith cards. I seem to have come full circle.

COVID continues to come under control nationally with fewer and fewer cases and deaths being reported. This is likely from a combination of the relatively speedy vaccine rollout over the last few months with some contribution of natural immunity due to the roughly 10-15% of the population that caught and recovered from the disease.

The health system is breathing easier. There are reports of COVID units with no patients for the first time in well over a year.

Does this mean we're done? I don't think so.

It's not a US disease; it's a global disease. We are still at the mercy of trends and problems of other regions—what happens in them regarding vaccine, and in the spread of variants with possible higher levels of contagion and higher mortality.

India continues to be a problem spot.

The official numbers there are echoing those here at the height of the winter surge this past January, but the excess mortality there is much higher (and woefully under-reported). Their official statistics only count those who die in a hospital with a positive COVID test. Those who die at home, or those who die waiting for care, who have not yet been tested, are not counted.

Here in Alabama, we seem to have more or less reached the limit of the easily vaccinated. A measly 35% of the population has at least one vaccine; only 28% are fully vaccinated. Demand has fallen off. The large vaccination centers are closing one by one despite the huge number of residents who could still benefit.

We're a few percentage points higher locally in Jefferson county, but we remain at risk with about a 4.5% positivity rate on tests and between 6 and 7 cases per 100,000 population daily.

On my wanderings through life this past week, I noticed that people are still masking up when going indoors in public places but generally wearing them under their noses which defeats the whole purpose. Can we get those numbers up? Only with some massive public health campaigns to counter some of the more ridiculous propaganda that has spread. I doubt any of our state or local agencies have the funds or the energy for that. Our local mask ordinance expires in another week and probably won't be continued.

I'm not worried about myself at this point. Nor am I overly worried about most of my patients. They fought tooth and nail to find vaccine when it first came out. As elders, they understood they were at much higher risk.

The CDC guidance is likely to keep evolving so that the vaccinated will be given free run of society while the unvaccinated will be told to continue to use caution and restraint. This is going to result in a sort of society-wide honor system regarding masks which isn't likely to be terribly helpful. After all, the great American public was hoarding gasoline in plastic garbage bags only two weeks ago. There's going to be no way to know if the maskless are vaccinated or simply deranged.

My rules are: no need to mask outdoors; and no need to mask with a small group of friends who are vaccinated; mask in a store or other place with a lot of people I don't know. Health facilities are likely to continue the masking rule for quite some time as it has cut down quite a bit on disease transmission of all stripes. I'll continue to wear one at work for the indefinite future, at least while I am working in clinical care.

><

I went out last night (masked) to one of the first performances at the new Red Mountain Theater Arts Campus that's taken shape near the ballpark: a table read of a new script about the history of lynchings in Jefferson County that acts as both exploration of the real lives of the people and a memorial to them and condemnation of the heinous acts perpetrated upon them.

The evening featured a powerhouse cast, many of whom I have known for years or have worked with on a project or two. The author took historical research and his imagination to intertwine the stories, the social trends that created the conditions that allowed for lynching to happen, and, as with all good theater, a mirror for the audience to see themselves along with a litany of present-day names and incidents showing how the stains of the past continue to color the present. It has a great future as a theater piece, but it was so powerful in the simple way it was presented, that I worry that a wish to create a fully realized staging might lead to temptations to overproduce and lessen its impact.

><

I just finished Isabel Wilkerson's new book *Caste* which posits that the way in which we need to view American society is as a caste system, every bit as complex and rigid as the one in India, and that many of the difficulties of our times and much modern politics—everything from the white working-class consistently voting against their own economic interests to the poor response to the pandemic—can be explained by the thousand-and-one little social rules we unconsciously abide by to keep certain people in the ruling caste and other people locked into subordinate castes. I highly recommend it.

I am not a product of the Deep South, having not come here until my mid-30s. I have always been able to see certain things that I have considered wrong and called out which others have considered normal. But the more reading I have done, the more I have come to understand my own socialization and unconscious biases.

I have spent years trying to unlearn them and replace them with more equitable ways of viewing the world. This is a constant battle but it's a good fight. I hope my African-American friends see me continually working to improve.

Tommy, coming from a Walker County white working-class background, always accused me of having been born with a silver spoon. I suppose I was in some ways, but I've been trying to use it to dig my way to a better understanding of all of us.

WEDNESDAY | MAY 26, 2021

IT'S RAINING THIS EVENING. Church choir rehearsal, held outside, was cut rather short.

It's obvious that my fellow Unitarians did not grow up in Seattle. Those of us who did, learned at an early age to trudge forward with whatever outdoor activity is at hand whether water is falling from the skies or not.

I will admit that Southern rains can be, at times, real gully washers that make this attitude impractical, but tonight's has been a gentle rain, more like the drifting mists of home. I suppose the handling of soggy sheet music would have been unpleasant and we did get the pieces we needed to record for future services down so all was not lost.

It did not rain last night. I took a couple of friends out for our first fine dining meal in 15 months. Vino in Mountain Brook has a large outdoor patio, the weather was warm, and we enjoyed the whole gamut from cocktails to appetizers to mains to dessert. Good food, good friends, good conversation. I had almost forgotten that sort of activity existed. I had scallops in curried cream sauce. It's probably not on my diet plan and I know the tiramisu wasn't. I'll work on losing my pandemic 20 another day.

As the world starts to open back up, I, along with the rest of us, am trying to figure out what the rules should be regarding social distancing and mask use. All of our local mask ordinances expired as of Monday and are not being renewed, so we are all left with CDC guidelines (or misinterpretations thereof) and various corporate policies.

I am continuing with my policies in some situations and not in others based on what I think is a combination of common sense and good public health. I don't mind wearing a mask. I've gotten so used to it over the last year or so that I don't even notice when I have it on half the time. If it's not on, it rides around in my back pocket along with a spare just in case.

I work in health care which means I go in and out of buildings dedicated to healing and into which people with various illnesses, immune deficiencies, and other conditions that prevent them from being vaccinated at this time, congregate. Therefore, both UAB and the VA are continuing mask mandates in buildings used for clinical care for the foreseeable future.

We wear masks with patients, when in inpatient care areas, and when in the public areas of the building such as lobbies, hallways, and elevators. If we're in office suites or other places where patients do not go, we'll take them off as staff are all vaccinated.

I am still wearing mine indoors in buildings where I don't know others' health and vaccination status such as in stores. I think it's polite. It telegraphs that I give a damn about the health of my fellow citizens and the health of the employees in such establishments.

I don't wear it outside unless there's a crowd of people (like the Saturday morning farmers market). I don't wear it at home or when in the company of a few people who are all vaccinated. I do wear it on house calls as that's a healthcare situation.

If and when I start going back to the movies or getting on airplanes, I'll gladly wear it. COVID is not the only respiratory disease out there, and I've noted that I haven't had a single cold or bronchitis infection since this whole thing started. I usually get a couple a year.

❦

While things are definitely improving, this whole thing isn't over yet, not by a longshot.

There are still about 30 people in UAB hospital with active COVID infections and another 30 who are not actively infectious, but who are still too sick to go home. This is way down from the average of 300 a day we hit in January, but it's still a burden. Because the older population has been better about getting vaccinations, it's mainly younger and middle-aged people who are deathly ill.

Hospitalization rates for the vaccinated have fallen to negligible levels. Those few who get COVID infections post-vaccination generally don't develop complications that can't be handled at home. Hospitalization rates for the unvaccinated population really haven't changed.

It looks like nationally we're going to end up with about 60% vaccinated and 40% not by the Fourth of July. That 40%, as it's a younger and healthier cohort than the total population, won't have the roughly

2% chance of death we've seen; it will be lower. But, that population is so large that there is still the chance of thousands and thousands of excess deaths still to come from what is starting to become a preventable disease.

It's important to keep in mind that this doesn't account for the unknown long-term complications of the illness. There's lots of end organ damage noted in many studies. It might not matter much when you're 35, but it might play havoc a couple of decades later at 60 and shave years off of life expectancy.

We now have a truly ridiculous law in Alabama banning "vaccine passports" and not allowing public or private entities to discriminate regarding access to the public based on vaccine status. It's so inartfully written that it basically forbids state institutions, including UAB, from handing out vaccine documentation cards. Nor will it allow schools to ever add another vaccine requirement for students, no matter what diseases may be in circulation. It also tramples on the private property rights of individuals and businesses.

It's likely to be ignored for the most part, but could certainly pop up as a poison pill in the future when the next pandemic disease comes to town. And there *will* be a next one. If our grandparents had, in the 40s and 50s, acted as we are today, we'd still be battling polio and smallpox.

So do your civic duty and get your vaccine if you haven't yet done so. Operators are standing by to take your appointment. The folks at the CDC and WHO with their years of training in virology and epidemiology and their billion-dollar budgets are savvier than you and your Google search and your friends on Facebook.

MONDAY | MAY 31, 2021

I T'S BEEN A LONG WEEKEND.

It has felt like the first normal holiday weekend in a year-and-a-half, bookended as it was by backyard barbecues with old theater friends on Friday evening and again with another group earlier this evening. Good friends, good conversation, and the reliving of past triumphs and tragedies on the boards—the kind of reminiscing that theater people always do when they get together.

I've noticed that theater folk are pretty much the same, at least in the English-speaking world, with their referential quips to famous lines and lyrics, spontaneous sing-alongs, and stories of random mishaps both backstage and onstage. I haven't been to too many Broadway salons, but I imagine it's not all that different.

I completed a major project I set for myself this weekend. I got plants into all the pots on my deck so I could have some flowers and visual interest outside my windows. One trip to Home Depot for potting soil, several flats of annuals, a couple of hibiscuses, a rose bush, and a few other assorted odds and ends, and I have living growing things around my seating areas.

It remains to be seen if I can keep them alive for the season. I have two spots left. I've decided I'll get a couple of potted ornamental cypress trees for those areas. I've seen some nice ones for sale at the Botanical Gardens, so I'll make a trip over there this next week.

We're rapidly evolving into a two-tiered society of vaxxed and unvaxxed. People end up in one camp or the other for various reasons but, if you wish to get the vaccine, it's now available essentially anywhere to anyone over the age of 12.

The relatively quick distribution of the last few months has contributed to a sharp drop in cases and deaths back to what they were in the earliest stages of the pandemic more than a year ago. But they do continue to mount, fed by the significant percentage of the population that remains unvaccinated.

We're now at about 595,000 deaths in the US since the beginning of the pandemic, with only 15,000 to go before we surpass the Civil War to become the second greatest mass casualty event in US history. (The 1918 flu has the number one slot at 675,000 deaths.)

The rate of spread in the unvaccinated population remains roughly the same as it was at the height of the pandemic in January. Death rates are lower because the unvaccinated population tends to be younger and healthier. But there are still going to be a lot of people who die who don't need to because of lingering propaganda from a previous administration that has poisoned certain communities' trust in sound science.

When the variant from India, now named Delta, gets here (and it will get here) with its much higher levels of transmissibility, and makes its way into the unvaccinated population, we may find ourselves back to overburdened COVID wards and strained health systems.

It won't be as bad as this past year. We've figured out what we're doing in terms of treatment and we're better at keeping people alive, but I remain gravely concerned about the health effects we don't know about.

We've become familiar with the small percentage of long haulers who months later have significant viral symptoms, but I suspect there's end organ damage that's going to manifest in a decade or so as early-onset chronic kidney disease, or chronic obstructive pulmonary disease, or early-onset dementia, or congestive heart failure. This is going to take a lot of people, and the health system as a whole, by surprise.

I shall be happily retired at that point. I don't know when exactly I'll retire, but COVID has certainly pushed me towards earlier rather than later. The fact that it is sneaking up on me was brought home by my receipt of my retirement packet from the University of California system that arrived in the mail this past week.

My pension under that system stops accruing on my 60th birthday next year, so it makes no sense to not start taking it at that time. It won't amount to a lot of money but, considering what that system did to me and Steve, I plan on collecting every penny out of them I can. The best revenge is living well.

You may not have to wear a mask anymore if you're vaccinated, but it's still a good idea to wash your hands.

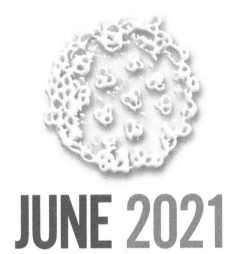

JUNE 2021

Anything Goes

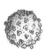

THURSDAY | JUNE 3, 2021

W E'RE ALMOST AT 600,000 DEATHS in the US from COVID. We're still having between 500 and 1,000 deaths daily, so we should pass that mark in another week. When we hit 610,000, and we will by the Fourth of July weekend, the pandemic will officially pass the Civil War to become the second-largest mass casualty event in US history.

The first is the 1918 flu pandemic at 675,000. I can see COVID passing that over the course of this year if we don't get better at reaching and reducing the unvaccinated population.

My inpatient friends tell me that there's still a significant number of people coming in with new COVID infections. They aren't coming in the numbers they were earlier this year, so the system is having no problems absorbing them.

They all have one thing in common: they hadn't gotten a vaccine. The inpatient docs are losing empathy for them as they are having to expend time and energy saving people from what is rapidly becoming a preventable disease.

The next big turning point is going to come when the FDA moves the vaccines from emergency use authorization (EUA) to approved status. I don't know when that's going to happen, but more than 120 million successful vaccinations in the US with minimal complications and side effects is a pretty compelling data set. As long as vaccines remain under EUA, they remain "experimental" and it's difficult to have regulations requiring them.

Approved vaccines, however, have plenty of laws backing the rights of employers, schools, and other entities to demand vaccination. Once that happens, it will be interesting to see what happens to the anti-vaccine forces. I also remain suspicious that once the vaccines have official FDA approval, there will be a push by the insurance industry to add riders to health policies denying payment of claims for COVID-19 treatment in the voluntarily unvaccinated.

>≈⊃

It's been a quiet work week chez Andy.

All the usual chores have been completed and the clinical programs for which I have responsibility are humming along without too much difficulty or need for excess oversight. It's rather a nice change.

I do chafe, however, at the amount of data entry that's now required of me. It seems to have doubled over the course of the pandemic.

One would think that the US healthcare system would prefer its physicians to act as doctors rather than as typists but I could be wrong. It reminds me of my days back in the 70s as a keypunch operator. (To my younger readers, google Hollerith cards).

Nothing new has turned up yet as far as the performance career goes. The local theaters are all starting to get people together to figure out how to move forward in our changed environment, so there should be projects I can audition for soon.

A couple of people have suggested that I take selections from these posts and turn them into a one-man Spalding Gray-type monologue for performance. I'm not absolutely against that idea, but I'd need an external director/dramaturg to help shape it properly. That's not something I think I could do. I don't have the correct objective eye for the material.

If someone thinks this is a brilliant idea and wants to work on it, I'm open to conversation. In the meantime, something will come along soon. It usually does. I have board meetings for the Opera and a theater company, and a focus group for another theater company in the next two weeks, so I should start to hear things.

I have been asked to participate as a storyteller in a local festival fundraiser next month. I have no idea why they asked me, but I foolishly said yes and now have to come up with a five to seven-minute piece.

The theme of the evening is apparently animals. I can't think of any of my personal stories involving animals that would keep an audience interested for that length of time. Perhaps my story that ends up with a glass Murano fish will do. (If you've heard me tell the story, you'll know what I'm referring to).

I had a very odd dream last night.

I was tasked with rescuing Queen Elizabeth from the top of some cliffs. I picked her up, tucked her under my arm, and scaled down a rocky escarpment that turned into an urban hellscape. Eventually, I had to grab a rope and swing with her across a chasm in true Luke and Leia fashion to get her back to Buckingham Palace.

Then, because I was wearing my pajamas, I had to go to the costume shop to find something appropriate to wear to the royal reception. There was nothing in my size other than mismatched plaids in neon colors.

Someone will have to explain this one to me. My major takeaway was that the 95-year-old queen wasn't very heavy, so I had no difficulty picking her up and having her cling to my side.

Perhaps it's my inner David Lynch coming out. I've been binge-watching *Twin Peaks*. I hadn't ever seen it. It came out in 1990 when I was in residency, working 80 hours a week and watching essentially no TV. I'd always heard about it, knew most of the references, but hadn't a clue what it was really about.

It's interesting to see the exteriors of the Pacific Northwest as it was in my youth, but I'm not sure I completely get the highly stylized performances and storytelling. If anything, it seems to be some sort of send-up of the overblown evening soaps of the 80s like *Dynasty* and *Falcon Crest*. I can see why it didn't last very long. Still, at least I'll now be able to say I've seen it.

One of the Broadway pages, in response to the Spielberg version of *West Side Story* that's due out shortly, was discussing pairing up other famous film directors with musical remakes. I suggested a David Lynch version of *Hello, Dolly!* It would be weirdly fascinating and likely more watchable than the film we have. I wonder if Sheryl Lee is available?

MONDAY | JUNE 7, 2021

WENT TO A MOVIE TONIGHT.

I think it's been nearly 18 months since I last set foot in a movie theater (and I can't even remember what film I saw on the big screen). It was a friend's birthday and his family rented out one of the theaters at The Summit multiplex for a group of vaccinated friends to enjoy.

The movie was Disney's new *Cruella*, an origin story for the villainess of *101 Dalmatians*. How was it? Better than it had any right to be with a fabulous costume/production design, a killer soundtrack, and a couple of great performances from the two Emmas, Stone and Thompson, as dueling malevolent fashion divas.

It's also 20 minutes too long, drags badly in the middle, and is way too sophisticated for most children unless your 8-year-old son is asking for an Auntie Mame Barbie for Christmas. MNM will write up her review later.

This is my second birthday party of the week. For the weekend, I made a mad dash to Columbia, South Carolina to attend the one-year delayed 50th (now 51st) 'birthday of a dear friend. I spent time with various Columbia theater luminaries, many of whom I have gotten to know through my forays into online performance over this last year. It was nice to finally meet some cast members in person.

My friend is an Anglophile. So cucumber sandwiches were consumed (they were available at the market for ready money), libations were imbibed, and it all ended up with a rather hilarious croquet match on the highly uneven and root-snagged back lawn played through the dusk and into the dark, necessitating portable lanterns to see whose ball was whose. I would not have been surprised to have seen a stray hedgehog or flamingo.

It's safe to say that vaccinated social life is starting to return to normal. In reading over the statistics, transmission rates in the states where vaccines have been readily accepted are way down along with a significant decline in hospitalization and death rates.

In states like mine, which has stalled out at about a 40% vaccination rate, numbers aren't necessarily going up but they aren't flatlining either as the virus continues to march through the willfully unvaccinated population.

So, while I think we are approaching the end of the acute phase of the pandemic, I don't think we're at the end of COVID by a long shot. It will continue to fester in susceptible populations. Some of those individuals, healthy teens through middle-aged adults, are going to become deathly ill. Some will die and there's no need for it.

It's a sad situation but I just don't know what I, or any one of us as individuals, can do at this point. I'm just waiting for the Delta variant from India to firmly establish itself in the US (it's going to get here) with its much higher levels of transmission. The vaccines seem to protect against it just fine, but it could start burning through the unvaccinated population at very rapid rates leading to a new surge just as we think we've got a handle on things. And it's going to happen in the states least equipped to handle another surge due to the weaknesses in health structure wrought by decades of right-wing austerity politics.

⚰️

I'm feeling worn out by the events of the last year-and-a-half.

I don't know if I'm crashing from a prolonged adrenaline high or am disillusioned by the realities of modern politics and healthcare policy. My mind keeps wandering to retirement and doing something else.

The pandemic has exposed the fault lines not just in how the medical system works, but also in my life. I haven't figured out yet whether it will be better to paper over the cracks or to wedge them open and break things apart so I can construct solutions in a new way.

My next big project, which I've been putting off for a year, is to go through all of my boxes of ephemera and family papers, and genealogical research that have accumulated over the decades. I'm the family archivist so it's all come to rest with me. I want to put it all in order and digitize what needs to be saved so it can be passed down in some semblance of a filing system to the next generation, assuming one of my nieces is going to be interested.

There's nothing on the theatrical calendar for the rest of the year yet. Something will turn up. It usually does. There are rumblings of a new edition of *Politically Incorrect Cabaret*. There are a couple of things in the wind for which I might audition. I'm going to have to go back to voice lessons before doing another musical; not singing much for a year-and-a-half hasn't helped my instrument in the least.

There are a number of board and planning meetings coming up with various theater groups I am involved with to try and shore up finances before venturing into production again. Will getting a juicy role to work on help my inner ennui? Maybe I just need a weekend at the beach. I'll solve it eventually. I always do.

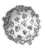

SATURDAY | JUNE 12, 2021

T OMORROW, THE US WILL HIT 600,000 COVID DEATHS since the beginning of the pandemic.

As the vaccines have rolled out and the educated moneyed classes have been protected, there's less and less interest in following the disease in real-time. State health departments are no longer uploading daily totals, but rather twice a week or even weekly totals. That may make the functionaries who gather and tabulate data have an easier life, but we lose the ability to pinpoint what's going on with any accuracy.

These decisions are being made just as the Delta variant, which spreads much more quickly than the original strain, is starting to make significant inroads and, with more lax data reporting, it's possible that weeks may go by before we start to notice a disturbing trend. And with exponential numbers, this may be a significant issue.

Today is either the 456th or the 458th day of the pandemic. It's the former if we use the date the Trump administration called a national emergency on March 13, 2020—two days after the WHO declared the SARS-2 coronavirus a global pandemic on March 11.

Thanks to human ingenuity, and some political changes at the top, things are starting to return to normal, at least among the privileged classes with access to vaccines, health care, information, communication, transportation, and all the rest of it.

Those of us who live in this world usually consider it to be the norm as everyone they know and interact with on any sort of equal footing belongs to it. I spend a good part of my life, thanks to decades of house calls and case management programs, in rural and impoverished areas, in and out of the homes of people who are not of this world.

For various reasons, the pandemic isn't over there and isn't likely to be over there for quite some time. One of the great failings of our health system currently is that it's designed by the upper classes for the upper classes.

There are really no mechanisms by which less privileged communities can get in on the ground floor to tell their stories so that systems can be designed to help them from the ground up rather than through shoddy attempts at retrofitting after the fact.

A great case in point was the pivot to telemedicine last spring where more than one health administrator of my acquaintance assumed that all patients would have a smartphone or iPad, home WiFi, and be adept at using said tools.

We hit 100,000 domestic deaths on 5/27/2020 (Day 77). 200,000 on 9/22/2020 (Day 195). 300,000 on 12/14/2020 (Day 278). 400,000 on 1/19/2021 (Day 314). 500,000 on 2/22/2021 (Day 348), and now 600,000 on 6/13/2021 (Day 458). Obviously, the vaccine is working to reduce the death toll but the disease remains. Anecdotally, it's circulating mainly in unvaccinated populations where, as the substrate tends to be young and healthy, it's not causing the same rates of illness.

However, it continues to send people who should have long and fruitful lives ahead of them to the ICU and from there to the morgue. As more than half of the state of Alabama remains unvaccinated, despite the pleading of all of us who work in health care, we're going to be coping with COVID for a very long time.

Today was Central Alabama Pride. Given the pandemic conditions of the last year, planning and permitting for the usual parade in Birmingham was not possible, so it was more of a street fair with entertainment this year. It was hot and sticky so I didn't stay long, but I did break out my festive new shirt bought for the occasion covered with rainbow dragons.

I do so like to be tastefully understated in my sartorial choices. In my 40-plus years as an adult gay man (most of them very out of the closet), I have been to lots of Pride celebrations.

I've been to parades and gatherings in Seattle, Sacramento, San Francisco, Los Angeles, San Diego, Birmingham, Atlanta, New York, and Amsterdam—and those are just the ones I can recall quickly. I have rainbow T-shirts, necklaces, hats, and other accouterments stretching back to the mid-80s packed away in various boxes.

Steve, who loved Pride because he came out seven years prior to Stonewall, and had way too many memories of police raids and a complete inability to be an authentic human in public, instilled the value of Pride celebrations in me during our years together. It was one day where we could walk down the street, hand in hand, without fearing reprisals. Where we could greet friends with a hug and a peck on the lips without drawing withering stares.

Wherever we were in June, we made sure to attend the local celebration. My standard uniform for Pride for years was a T-shirt he bought me at San Francisco Pride, our first summer together, with a hand-done silkscreen of a rainbow over the Golden Gate Bridge.

The Prides of the 80s and early 90s of my youth were very different than they are now. LGBTQIA issues were not part of the national conversation. There were no corporate sponsors. (The liquor companies and HIV pharmaceutical companies started to creep in in the 90s sometime.) Everything was local community time and energy.

The moneyed gay community, at best discreetly out, did not make free with their power and connections. Things were a bit ramshackle, but the HIV crisis had turbocharged the need to organize and to get things done quickly and efficiently. This spilled over into Pride and didn't just reside in health care.

Young people of today have no idea of how different it was—the presence of the sick among us, the inability of public officials to recognize the existence of the community, the knowledge that if the wrong person spotted you, even as an observer on the sidewalk, that it could mean the loss of your job or your lease. Now Target hauls out the rainbow merchandise in June in the annual rotation between Easter and the Fourth of July. A whole new world indeed.

Tommy was deeply ambivalent about Pride. He was fine with the concept and would usually go with me to the event, but he didn't like the fact that the most visible parts would be the drag queens or the leather guys or the go-go boys from the local strip bar. He hated that those images dominated the media coverage and that the world would then apply those images to him.

I kept trying to explain to him that we live in a visual media world and that whatever makes the best visuals is going to make the news. You don't get ratings when you broadcast a bunch of gay and lesbian CPAs walking down the street in business suits. He would have none of it.

I don't mind any of it. It's our party. We can act and dress how we want. It doesn't make us less human or less worthy of respect. The straight world is perfectly welcome to join the party but it's the one day a year that it gets to be our day and our rules, and if you don't like it, you can lump it.

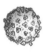

TUESDAY | JUNE 15, 2021

'M RETURNING TO THE FIELD with my VA house call program. Today was spent in Huntsville, last Thursday in Guntersville, and shortly off to Jasper. If all goes according to plan, I will be adding Childersburg to the list. At that point, if we can get functional teams in Muscle Shoals and Anniston, we'll be able to offer house calls to every veteran in the Birmingham VA catchment area.

If I retire with that having been accomplished, I'll have managed to do something lasting with my job. Hopefully, the stars will align. Who am I kidding? It's not up to the stars, it's up to the bean counters in a back-office making decisions based on allocated funding and cost-benefit analyses.

Medicine, like everything else in US society, revolves entirely around money. The first thing I teach medical students when they ask why things are a certain way is for them to figure out who is being paid and how much. That usually answers their question for them.

I don't have much to report from Covidland.

We are over the 600,000 death mark. Only 10,000 more to go to top the Civil War in terms of casualties. We'll likely hit that by fall as we're still recording dozens, if not hundreds of deaths each day.

The rates around here, which had been falling precipitously through the spring thanks to vaccination, have stalled and are now inching back up due to the number of unvaccinated people in our local communities. While many states are celebrating the 70% level, Alabama remains stalled around 40%.

The number of vaccines given the last couple of weeks has been going up, possibly due to the end of school and more free time for people to go get one, but we still need a lot more. We're now about two weeks out from the long Memorial Day weekend. The hospitalization rate, if it's been affected by behavior changes, should reflect that this next week or so. The death rate will reflect it the first couple of weeks of July.

I've run into a number of people recently who have developed COVID these last few weeks despite being fully vaccinated. I'm wondering if that's the spread of the more contagious and virulent Delta variant.

The good news is that studies and anecdotal evidence have shown that if you catch the disease after full vaccination, you may be miserable for a while, but you won't be sick enough to require hospitalization and the chance of death is negligible.

The bad news is that as people jettison their masks and learned behaviors for "normal", while more than half remain unvaccinated, your chance of running into the disease remains rather high and, as the Delta variant takes hold and aggressively crowds out other strains, you may get sick this summer. I don't take foolish chances, but I'm fully cognizant that I am not immune to the vagaries of fate, so I'm expecting to feel rotten sometime between now and Labor Day.

The big thing at work, as far as my patients go, has been the approval of aducanumab (trade name Aduhelm), the first new medication for Alzheimer's disease in decades. There has been some breathless coverage in the lay press aimed at seniors, which has got a lot of people worked up about a potential miracle drug for themselves or loved ones.

Alzheimer's disease is one of the scariest diseases out there for most elders. Everyone recognizes it as the disease that destroys the self and, as the self is the most basic concept we have in Western thought, it is absolutely devastating for all involved. I'm rehearsing my speeches for my patients in my head so when they ask, I can let them down gently and explain that the drug is not what they think it is. Most drugs rarely are.

When I entered geriatrics, back in the very early 1990s (30 years ago next month), there were no real medical treatments for Alzheimer's or other dementias. We tried to control symptoms with various psychoactive drugs, often not very well, but we experimented and learned and stopped doing some of the more destructive things we were doing at the time because we didn't know any better.

Actually, there was one drug on the market for dementia—hydergine. I don't think they even make it anymore as it didn't work. Everyone knew that the major mechanism in memory involved neurons using acetylcholine as a neurotransmitter. The thought was that if you could increase the amount of that chemical in the brain, things would get better. The problem is that taking oral acetylcholine is useless as gastric acid breaks it down into acetate and choline which get nowhere near the brain.

People were experimenting with direct injections of acetylcholine into brain ventricles and all sorts of other iffy things without much success until someone hit on the idea of just using the acetylcholine that was already in the brain. Rather than adding more, create a medicine that would prevent it from being broken down in the brain's constant recycling of materials.

Drugs were developed that blocked the enzyme responsible for this breakdown. The first one was tacrine (Cognex) which came out toward the end of my fellowship. It was imperfect. It had to be taken four times a day and it was very toxic to the liver in certain individuals, requiring regular blood tests. (Both of these things can be problematic in the demented.)

A few years later, better drugs came along with the same mechanism of action: donepezil (Aricept), rivastigmine (Exelon), and galantamine (Razadyne). They were not toxic in the same way and could be dosed once or twice a day.

None of these drugs is great. They may slow down the disease process some for a time, generally not more than a year or two, but they cannot prevent the disease's inexorable march across the brain. They are something, however, and we use them routinely.

About 20 years ago, one more drug appeared, memantine (Namenda). It has a very different mechanism of action. It prevents neural cell death by blocking the process of apoptosis—programmed cell destruction. It is only proven to have positive clinical effects in moderate dementia (the point at which someone cannot go into the bathroom in the morning and get ready for the day without help) but again, it's something.

Aducanumab, unlike these other medications, is not an oral drug but rather a monoclonal antibody that enters the brain and prevents amyloid protein (which slimes over and prevents proper function of neurons) from attaching itself and accumulating with time the way it usually does in Alzheimer's.

Clinical trials showed no clinical benefit in terms of improving memory in test subjects but did show a decline in protein accumulation over time. Whether this change manifests itself as any sort of benefit in a living person remains unclear.

This is why a lot of experts in the area were against the approval of the drug. A number of people affiliated with the FDA resigned when it was approved as they were so against a drug of such unclear benefit being launched on the world.

Monoclonal antibodies must be given as infusions, not as pills. They would be destroyed by the acid environment of the stomach. There are some significant brain bleeding complications in certain individuals requiring routine MRI scans of the brain to detect early problems.

Trying to explain infusions and MRIs to the demented can be problematic and the procedures themselves are scary. Then there's the cost. Biogen has decided that $56,000 a year is appropriate. It is unclear which insurances are likely to cover it due to its weak evidence. The FDA has demanded post-approval data showing clinical benefit or they will rescind their approval. We don't know if it will be possible to ascertain this.

Needless to say, it's not high on my list of things to prescribe. I've been laying this all out to patients and families so they have information on which to base choices. We'll see who opts for the drug, and I'll report back on my clinical experience when I have some.

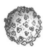

SATURDAY | JUNE 19, 2021

HAPPY JUNETEENTH. (A holiday long-deserved which better not be taken over by white culture with mattress sales or beer busts.)

Mine is starting at 4:30 AM. It's my call weekend and a resident at the nursing home that I cover as part of my call duties decided this was the right time to act up in such a way that the nurses needed to wake me up.

Call is a necessary part of the job and my duties aren't especially onerous (about three weeknights a month and a weekend every other), but I learned long ago that my brain/sleep physiology is such that if I'm woken up in the middle of the night, I rarely am able to get myself back to sleep again, and I'll be faced with a number of hours of wakeful tiredness before I have to get up and face whatever the next day has to bring.

This is my first call night without a beeper. UAB has finally fully joined the digital/cell phone age and replaced beepers with an app on our smartphones that serves a similar function. Having had a beeper on my belt for professional purposes for something over 30 years, it feels odd to be without one.

I was a bit worried that the phone wouldn't wake me up. (I'm well-conditioned to that obnoxious beep but can sleep through nearly anything else—internship, in the pre-limitations on residency work hours, will do that to you.) However, the ringtone they've chosen is piercing enough to work just fine. So here I am, in the pre-dawn hours, listening to the birds outside my bedroom window greeting the imminent arrival of the miracle of another day and batting away Anastasia who is trying to help me type.

The persistence of the beeper is only part of the healthcare system's continued reliance on 80s/90s technology. For instance, we are the only industry that still runs on the fax machine as an essential mode of communication. I still have a landline not because I use it or because anyone ever actually calls me on it but because it's necessary at times for me to fax documents larger than the fax app on my smartphone can handle.

Some of this is due to the medico-legal system. Most of the laws that govern the handling of medical information were written 40 or 50 years ago and haven't been updated to take modern technology into account. Things change piecemeal bit by bit. The electronic transfer of prescriptions for controlled substances, which used to only be valid via hardcopy with an original signature, became a reality a couple of years ago making everyone's lives easier.

The home care and hospice industries, however, still run on fax, and I get about 150 pages a week, each of which needs to be signed and dated and sorted into the appropriate piles to fax back.

Everything in the medical system requires the signature of a licensed physician somewhere on some piece of paper in order for things to move forward. (Electronic signatures now work within certain parts of electronic health records). If we were all to break our wrists on the same weekend, the entire US healthcare system would grind to a halt.

Some of the lack of progress comes from the inherent conservatism of the profession and its practitioners. You don't really learn to be a physician in medical school. You learn a lot of random facts and you learn how to train your mind to sort through those facts and parse them properly to understand what's going on. All the things you really need to know are actually learned on the job by observing your colleagues and peers and modeling what they do.

This makes the profession very dependent on "We do it that way because we've always done it that way" thinking. It's highly resistant to change that does not naturally enter the workflow through physician practice.

If you ever want to see physicians, especially clinicians, get their collective backs up, try imposing mandates on what they do from outside—especially when they come from areas where they are designed by individuals who are not themselves practicing clinicians.

Then there are the silos and fractures in the system regarding information. Every other country with an advanced health system has a single way of collecting data and recording patient information no matter where in the system you may go. This allows charts to be shared electronically between any physician or nurse, any hospital, or any ancillary service with everyone working off a single data stream.

We have this in our country in just one place—the VA system.

It's possible to pull up the same records in any VA hospital or clinic from Fairbanks to Miami. Everywhere else in the US works off jealously guarded proprietary information systems which do not interface with each other.

I can see everything that happens in the UAB system in a patient's electronic chart but if they see a provider or obtain a service outside of UAB, even if it's across the street, forget it. (Unless somebody sends a fax.)

Patients and their families really don't understand this issue. They think that records miraculously move from place to place. A huge amount of my time is spent trying to reconstruct what happened in another emergency room or repeating a test I really didn't have to repeat because I had no way of accessing the results.

Even in the same institution, the data systems often don't interface properly. Often, the billing system and the clinical system don't talk to each other. This requires everything to be entered twice. It's why you're constantly filling out forms at the doctor asking for the same information over and over and over again.

We could have a single data system for health care in this country. It's been proposed countless times. It tends to be shot down for the same reasons that the rest of our infrastructure is falling apart. The only entity that's big enough to marshal the resources to make it work and bring it to every healthcare provider would be the federal government necessitating a large outlay of tax dollars and some sort of federal agency to run it.

For 40 years now, the more conservative of our political parties has run on a platform that government is the problem, not the solution. It wants all such issues handled through private enterprise. The result is many small private solutions, developed piecemeal to the detriment of the system and the health of the American public. It's not a problem I have a solution to as long as that philosophy remains entrenched.

Back to the beeper.

They have changed some over the years. When I started in medicine, they were analog shortwave radio receivers. In the hospital, you called a number, spoke into the phone, and your voice would emerge from the beltline of one of your colleagues. Given the age of medical residents and the punchiness of constant sleep deprivation, this usually led to a lot of practical jokes which we would find hilarious.

One female resident of my acquaintance announced that her beeper must be like a penis. It hung at the front of her pants and would call attention to itself at inopportune moments in an obnoxious manner. No one disagreed.

By the early 90s, beepers went fully digital and voices were replaced with short bursts of text. The arrival of the World Wide Web meant that you could access them from any digital device on your own. Before that, outside of the hospital, you had to call the hospital operator and ask them to access the system for you.

The hospital operators knew everything about everyone, and you never wanted to get on their bad side for fear they might spill the tea. The ones at UC Davis during my residency years were all very sweet and were good at keeping our private lives private—most of the time.

Digital communication has been a wild ride over my career—from landlines and payphones to car phones to cell phones to smartphones. You have to wonder what's next. Implantable devices allowing us to communicate with anyone anywhere without having to actually have an object external to our bodies? Wave your arm over the grocery check out to pay for your items? Download any piece of information directly into your brain? Who knows?

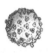

WEDNESDAY | JUNE 23, 2021

TODAY IS APPARENTLY INTERNATIONAL WIDOW(ER)S DAY. (The things you learn from social media.)

It hasn't quite become a Hallmark holiday yet. I suspect that even Hallmark would have difficulty selling greeting cards emblazoned with some variation of "Happy Widowhood!" on them.

It's not something one really feels like celebrating. It's just an uncomfortable fact of life when you have a partnership. If it ends through natural causes, as most do, one is going to survive the other. It's a state I can't really recommend.

The hardest part about it is no longer having that one other person who knows all your secrets and stories and shared memories. You can build a new life and new patterns, but the keeper of the flame of the old one is gone, the light is out in the temple, and later you start to wonder what was real and what was nostalgia as the partnership recedes into the mists of time with no one to help with a reality check.

Steve will have been gone 20 years six weeks from now. So much of our time together is almost dreamlike as we spent nearly all of it in another state, and I don't have a lot of contact with people who knew him on a regular basis.

Tommy, having been gone only three years, is much more real. There's a lot of life and many people around who knew and loved us as a unit, but I know even that will eventually change.

I'm thinking about the hundreds of thousands of new widows and widowers created over the last 15 months by the pandemic. At least mine happened during relatively normal times when I could be surrounded by people, have proper wakes/memorials, take the time I needed to travel, and do the things I know that help heal myself.

Too many people this year lost a partner to a plague they knew was allowed to spread through governmental inaction. They could not be present for the death. They could not hold a proper memorial. They had to retire immediately to the place of their memories. There was nowhere else for them to go. Just one more piece in the giant pile of mental health issues that COVID is leaving in its wake.

As the pandemic wanes and patterns return, those of us in health care are seeing upticks in behavioral issues: depression, anxiety, maladaptive coping mechanisms, and all the other frustrating and agonizing parts of the human condition. It's going to be a long few years and it's going to take a lot more than prescriptions for Zoloft and Ativan.

><&

We're at about 603,000 dead as of today.

The bodies are no longer piling up by the thousands, only by the tens and twenties, but it's still too many. With successful vaccines, COVID is essentially a preventable disease. Almost nobody has to die going forward but with about 35% of the population unvaccinated nationwide (closer to 60% in Alabama), the casualties will continue to mount.

There are now reports of the Delta variant in numerous places as hot spots are developing in communities with low vaccination rates. Rural Missouri appears to be spiking currently.

With Delta's increased transmissibility, increased virulence, and rapid spread among young and healthy people, there are going to be a lot more young widows and widowers in the coming weeks. Someone is going to have to explain to me why "freedom" is more important than "life" in the minds of those who are of a more conservative bent than I am. I just don't understand.

><&

I have the long weekend off and I thought perhaps a trip to the beach might be nice. Then I checked the lodging prices. When Motel

6 is over $400 a night, I stay home.

I'm assuming that the owners of lodging establishments are attempting to cash in on everyone's need for busting out of their cocoons of the last year-and-a-half, but I'm not sure predatory capitalism is the solution for society's current ailments. I foresee a lot of people running up some significant debt as they splurge and then having to try and service that debt in uncertain times. The 1918-19 pandemic helped fire off the Roaring 20s a century ago and we all know how that ultimately turned out for everyone in 1929.

I haven't told a story for a bit.

Here's one from a few years ago. Those of you who know me well know I have a bit of a weird GI system (Thanks for those genes, Dad) which can act up from time to time. Generally, it's under reasonable control with medication but if it decides to go crazy, there's not much I can do about it.

One of the things it can do is go into acutely painful intestinal spasm. I've gotten used to it—given that it's been happening since I was a teenager—but my autonomic nervous system never has. When it really gets going, it sends my parasympathetic nerves into overdrive which does various things, especially dropping my blood pressure, causing me to roll up my eyes and faint.

During medical school, I once did this in a room with 40 medical students and eight attendings. There was a great deal of clamor and I got a free tour of the emergency department on a stretcher.

The last time I had a severe attack, I was out shopping for supplies for one of Tommy and my famous cast parties. I had made the rounds—Winn Dixie, Sam's Club, and, as a last stop, the liquor store. As I headed up to the cashier with my bottles of Cointreau and Amaretto, it hit and, while waiting to pay my bill, down I went in an ashen heap much to the consternation of the cashier and the other patrons.

I came to enough to finish my transaction and stumble out the door. I just needed to get to the safety of my car. And down I went again in the rain in the middle of the parking lot. (Fortunately, the bottles did not break).

This time, I did not come to quickly and the ABC store clerk called the police about a drunk and disorderly. I was woken up by a nice policeman, was coherent enough to explain that I was a doctor, I was not drunk, I was not stoned, and I knew exactly what was happening. He took me at my word but flatly stated that he wasn't going to let me drive anywhere.

I returned home in the back of the squad car. I got home, took a nap, and then had to explain to Tommy, once he got home, just why we had to go back to the liquor store to pick up my car. He was greatly amused. Every time we went to the liquor store together after that, he would inquire innocently if he should catch me as we approached the register

It's missing the little jokes like that which can make widowhood difficult.

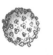

SUNDAY | JUNE 27, 2021

'VE BEEN EXHAUSTED MOST OF THE WEEKEND.

There's no reason for me to be particularly tired but I still slept ten hours Friday night, required a two-hour nap Saturday afternoon, slept another eight hours last night, and napped again today.

This reminds me of coming home from college for vacation. I'd do little but sleep as my body unwound from the stress of the previous quarter and prepared for the stress of the upcoming quarter.

I'm not sure if this is about the receding of COVID and political stressors, or if my body knows on some level that there's more to come and it's making me slow down and store energy for the next round. All I know is that I'm not proceeding terribly quickly on my next few projects.

Fortunately, they aren't things with specific deadlines attached, so if I keep losing time to naps, I'll still be OK. If nothing else, the cats seem very taken with my predilection for falling asleep, and snuggle up to do the same.

Covidland is relatively quiet.

The number of US deaths has dropped below 300 a day, despite the spread of the Delta variant. Whether this is now the new normal or the calm before the storm of an exponential rise in cases in states with low rates of vaccination remains to be seen.

The problem with exponential numbers is that everything seems placid and calm, and then all of a sudden things are everywhere seemingly out of the blue. It's entirely possible that there will be a relatively rapid rise in cases to be followed by increased mortality later this summer. We shall see what we shall see.

In the meantime, I'm taking advantage of a more open social life as the theater folk are starting to get back together now that we have all been vaccinated. There was a very nice backyard gathering last night where I saw many folk I have not seen for the last year-and-a-half.

><

As I don't really have much to say this evening, I suppose it's storytime. This one is from many decades ago, back when Steve and I were first together.

As I related in my last post, I have a bit of an odd GI tract that does weird things. One of the things that it does is react strangely to local water systems.

I figured this out years and years ago when every time I would visit LA, I would have an upset stomach that would go away as soon as I returned to Seattle or Northern California. I don't know what it is about LA, but I assume it has something to do with the mineral content of the water or how it's treated.

Steve was an LA boy who had only moved up to the Sacramento area about a year before we got together. Most of his friends remained in LA. We, therefore, drove down a couple of times a year to see some of his old friends and visit his old haunts. The run from Sacramento to LA down I-5 was about seven hours, so we could even bop down for a long weekend, especially with two drivers.

One visit, early in our relationship, we decided to go to Universal Studios. Neither of us had been for at least a decade and we thought it might be fun. We got up early to get to the gates before things opened so we wouldn't have to wait in line.

My upper GI tract was bothering me, as it usually did in LA, so I hadn't had any breakfast and really wasn't interested in eating anything. Steve was having none of it so he went over to the snack kiosk and bought me a banana and stood over me forcing me to eat it.

Ten minutes later, my stomach rebelled. The banana was threatening to reappear. We were in the middle of the plaza in front of the gates with no convenient restroom, so I did the only thing I could do and leaned over the rail at the edge. There was a drop of some 40 feet down to a flower bed to which the regurgitated banana sailed down, much to the consternation of the tourists marching up the drive.

Steve was mortified.

I felt much better and we ended up having a great time on the tour. Steve learned his lesson. Ever after, if I told him I wasn't hungry or didn't want to eat something, he took me at my word.

To this day, I don't eat bananas other than the occasional slice in a fruit salad. And don't get me started on banana pudding which is a staple of Alabama cuisine and constantly offered but always politely refused.

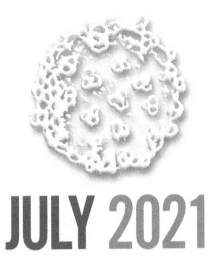

JULY 2021

Just One of Those Things

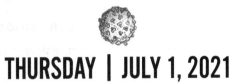

THURSDAY | JULY 1, 2021

I T'S ANOTHER MONTH and we're halfway through 2021.

At times, the days fly by. At other times, each one seems to drip, drip, drip by at an interminable pace. Pandemic thinking and experiences seem to have screwed up my brain's inner understanding of time. It no longer seems to be uniform with each hour identical. It's more elastic, stretching or compressing like Silly Putty, depending on events or inner moods.

❧

Society, at least around here, seems hell-bent on restoring itself as if the pandemic were over and there's a need to make up for lost time.

The problem is that it's not.

The number of cases and the death rate continue to inch up. We're at something over 605,000 dead now, not that much further until it surpasses the Civil War and becomes the second-largest mass casualty event in American history—the 1918-19 flu epidemic is likely to hold on to the number one spot, at least for a while.

The big problem area at the moment is Southwest Missouri, home of the Ozarks and Branson.

I would venture to guess that the latter is why this region has become the first major cluster of the Delta variant. The usual tourist traps are booming as people come out of a year or so of restricted life and movement. They have come from all over, crowded into various theaters and attractions, and brought their viral hitchhikers with them, passing them on to employees who then carry them into the surrounding communities.

The local hospitals are inundated again and transferring patients to St Louis and Little Rock. I have a feeling that this is a canary in the coal mine moment and, as visitors to the area return to their homes, Delta will soon be popping up in a community near you where, given its increased transmissibility over the original strains and its predilection for young and unvaccinated people, numbers will start rising in hospital systems elsewhere.

Given the usual timelines between seeding of the virus, a significant population developing virus, and when that population starts getting seriously ill, I'm thinking we'll start seeing a spike in casualties at the end of the month.

Of course, the vaccine will help, but the lack of enthusiasm for vaccination by a majority of the unvaccinated crowd means that even if it becomes clear that numbers are going up, the mass vaccination sites have been dismantled due to waning interest. There is roughly a month delay between first jab and full immunity, so they would have to begin the process now to be protected by August when we're likely to start seeing more concerning numbers.

I don't have a lot of empathy for willful anti-vaxxers who are becoming ill at this point.

Who I do have empathy for are the burnt-out healthcare workers who are being called on to keep on keeping on in a preventable situation. This has very real consequences.

People are quitting clinical healthcare positions in droves and there aren't a lot of folk standing in line to take their place. Almost everyone I know of my generation and older is taking a fresh look at their retirement plans.

The stories of docs having to not only do their work, but pitch in to change the sheets, administer the medications, and mop the floors due to a shortage of other clinical workers, are legion. Most physicians I know will buckle down and do anything necessary in a crisis, but it's not a sustainable long-term model for a functional health system.

I wish I had a better read at the moment on the business of healthcare.

From what I can tell, there's a major acquisition spree going on in the C-suites with small and medium-size players being swallowed up for larger interstate players. This seems to be true in most sectors of the business.

The AMA released a report this week that, for the first time, a majority of physicians worked for a hospital or health system entity rather than for themselves in private practice. I don't think that's necessarily a bad thing.

I have always worked for a large academic health system as faculty. It's a model I grew up with, it allows me a certain amount of freedom to feed my intellect and my soul as well as make money, and I like knowing how much money is coming in each paycheck.

I haven't gotten rich doing it, but I keep the bills paid and can afford to retire when I think the time is right. The problem is that most of the big players are not academic health systems, which are not-for-profit public goods, but rather private companies whose only goal, ultimately, is profit.

As the profit motive has invaded sector after sector of our economy and our lives, there's been a certain level of degradation of our way of living. The wheels of capitalism grind on, lifting a few up and right over the backs of most of the rest. When we are asked to choose profit or people, we currently choose profit and turn a blind eye to the people that the creation of profit may harm.

In medicine, the profit motive at upper levels leads to additional layers of byzantine bureaucracy as each tiny kingdom attempts to minimize its cost centers and buff up its balance sheet. It leads to clinicians being asked to do more and more with less support. (Support salaries are expensive).

This leads to an obsession with data and numbers rather than overall patient well-being. I keep having to teach medical residents that lab numbers are not interchangeable with the patient. Frequently, I'll ask that residents go talk to him or her and get a decent history about how they're feeling and what symptoms they're having before relying on what spits out of a lab computer.

The sucking of money out of systems for profit is leading to other problems as well. Compare our decayed public infrastructure with that in other wealthy countries and our political system that is having extreme difficulties coming up with solutions because they might require additional public spending.

It's seeping over into private spending as well. Would the Surfside condominium tower have collapsed if the squabbling residents in the HOA had been willing to fund the urgently needed repairs when they were identified several years ago?

Perhaps a few readers may be busy calling me a communist in their heads. I'm not. I'm just not a vulture capitalist who believes that everything should always be about profit all the time. The profit motive is a good one. It keeps us industrious. But I think it has to be shaped and managed by good government and policy, so that a handful of families don't control more wealth than half the country.

My work on rural house calls takes me into the homes of those whom capitalism has completely crushed through no fault of their own. I see a lot more of the downsides than most in the professional classes who have minimal contact with others not like themselves.

I've been booked as a "celebrity" storyteller at a fundraising event in a few weeks. I'm trying to decide just which of the stories of my life I need to tell. I'm leaning towards the saga of Steve's cremains as it's a classic, but I'm afraid it may be just a bit morbid. I should probably think of something a bit more uplifting.

While perusing the Internet this week, I found that a previous blog (written in December of 2005) is still online and accessible. Maybe I should poke around that.

I have had two other blog lives: one from 2001 started just after Steve died. I kept it going, off and on, through meeting Tommy in 2003 Sadly, I can't find a trace of it on the Internet, although it may be archived somewhere; I haven't taken the time to look yet.

I also contributed to a group blog called *Eternity LTD* from the late 1990s that covered the period where everything fell apart in California, and Steve and I had to relocate to Alabama. (I think I know where that one may have an archive.)

Do I dare read any of them?

Will I even be able to read these current posts in another decade without cringing? And what about the book I've written and this one to follow? Am I going to look at these in a few years as a significant accomplishment or a slight embarrassment?

I would like to think that practice is making my writing better with time, but one never knows, does one?

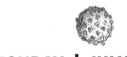

MONDAY | JULY 5, 2021

USUALLY, MONDAY IS MY DOUBLE-CLINIC DAY AT UAB. It's a slog through 14 or 15 patients with an emphasis on dementia, family dynamics, diabetes in poor control, the aftermath of strokes and heart attacks, and a few unsolvable social programs thrown in for good measure.

Thanks to the timing of the calendar, this Monday has been spent sleeping in, playing with cats, and carefully going through the first proof of Volume One of *The Accidental Plague Diaries,* page by page, to catch any errant typos or misprints that still remain. I'm about 40% through and have until next weekend to finish the job.

It feels strange and a little humbling to hold a physical copy of *The Accidental Plague Diaries* in my hands. I've always felt capable of writing a book but have never had the perseverance to take anything of this length to completion in the past.

As I reread it, yet again, trying to catch every last misplaced comma and minor spelling error, I'm torn between thoughts of "This is pretty good," and "This is three-hundred-and-some pages of navel-gazing."

I guess I'll just have to throw it out there into the world and see what the world ends up making of it.

The theme of the long weekend was social gatherings, both in-person and online: a game night at a friend's house; a Zoom game of Apples to Apples with a bunch of old friends from college now scattered around the country but with 40 years of shared history; and a 4th of July party that happens every year at an old friend's house which is one of the usual markers on the social calendar of Bohemian Birmingham. She lives right below Vulcan on Red Mountain and has a terrific view of the fireworks display.

As I stood there watching the explosions, my mind drifted back over various other fireworks celebrations I've attended over the years, some with family, some by myself, some with either Steve or Tommy at my side.

Steve was a Southern California boy who was the right generation to have come of age with Disneyland. He was seven when it opened and his parents took him opening week.

Steve and I went to Disneyland together many times during our California years. He always insisted that we stay until the end of the day for the fireworks. He took great joy in them, clapping and cheering as they carried him back to his childhood for a moment or two.

Tommy could take or leave fireworks but would stop what he was doing and enjoy them anytime they appeared. I remember standing on the back of a cruise ship with him as it pulled out of Nassau on the last night of the cruise that was our first vacation together, enjoying a fireworks display over the harbor arranged by Atlantis Events and being able to hold each other at the rail as we were in a safe gay space and could do that without fear of attack.

The most memorable fireworks I viewed alone were at the Tivoli Gardens in Copenhagen. The rules seem to be a bit different in Denmark. They were shot off so low to the ground that we could all feel the hot sparks drifting down on our scalps and cheeks. I found it a little unnerving.

✂

This weekend also marked the 40th anniversary of the first mention of what would come to be called the HIV epidemic in the press. It was a small article in the New York Times, appearing July 3, 1981, on page 20, taken from a mention in the *Morbidity and Mortality Weekly Report,* published by the CDC about a rare cancer (Kaposi's sarcoma) having been diagnosed in a cluster of gay men.

I didn't read it.

I was 19 at the time and not necessarily predisposed to reading the New York Times in a day before electronic accessibility. Even if I'd wanted to read it, I would have had a hard time finding a copy

I spent the summer of 1981 in the Bering Sea working on the University of Washington's oceanographic research vessel, the Thomas G. Thompson, running water sampling machinery on the graveyard shift. They weren't delivering a whole lot of New York papers then (or even now, I suppose) to Dutch Harbor in the Aleutians, the Pribilof Islands, Nunivak Island, or Seward on the Kenai peninsula.

I was busy punching buttons in the middle of the night, reading voraciously (I finished *War and Peace* in five days), and visiting the occasional elephant seal rookery. In the lower 48, natural and political forces were coming together that would end up shaping my life in ways I could not yet imagine.

I started to hear about the mysterious new disease when I got back to Stanford that fall (we were just down the peninsula from San Francisco), but I was still closeted. Beyond that, developing my dichotomous life between a double science major during the day, and a theater whiz in the evenings and weekends, didn't leave me a lot of time to get into too much trouble. This is the pattern that likely saved my life when so many others of my generation were taken.

As time went on and the negligence of the government condemned many in the gay community to death (shades of our current pandemic), I braced myself for a short life span and became determined to pack as much into it as I could, which is likely why I continue to overwork and over-commit. There's a piece of me that has been conditioned since my late teens to believe that there will never be enough time to complete my goals.

The biggest thing HIV ended up doing to me was killing off a majority of the out professional gay men a decade or so older than I. This meant that as I moved through my education and into my career, I had almost no gay role models. No mentors. No one who could help me navigate the inherent homophobia of academic medicine in the late 20th century. No one to help me open doors or smash glass ceilings. Consequently, I made more than a few mistakes over the years and my career took some unusual twists and turns.

It all came out OK, I think, but I sometimes wonder what I might have accomplished if HIV hadn't been a part of my times. It did, however, give me enough experience with how American society refuses to provide succor to marginalized populations in times of public health crisis to help me acquire some decent tools for handling my job over the years and to see many of the socio-political themes behind the current pandemic more clearly. If I couldn't do that, these essays, and the books that contain them, would not exist.

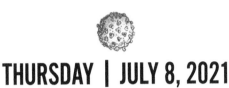

THURSDAY | JULY 8, 2021

YOU'D THINK BY NOW that I could start writing about something other than COVID. But the combination of Mother Nature's rules and human folly keep giving me grist for the mill.

Here are some statistics I've come across in the last few days.

First, the number of global deaths has topped 4 million. The United States continues to tick up, not at the rate seen six months ago but still ever upwards. We're at about 606,500 today.

Second, the cluster in Southern Missouri I alluded to earlier this week continues to explode with local hospitals swamped and EMS runs happening frequently per local news sources. The deaths will spike in two to three more weeks per the usual patterns.

Third, the percentage of Delta variant cases nationwide was running about 20% in mid-June. It increased to 30% at the end of that month and now, just over a week later, it's over 50%. Given its much more rapid transmissibility, it'll be over 90% by the end of the month.

Fourth, here in Jefferson county, the number of cases of COVID doubled this week over last week. The number of people hospitalized at UAB with COVID has grown five-fold from 5 to 25 in the past week.

What do all of these cases have in common? Lack of vaccination.

Somewhere between 94% and 99% of infections requiring significant medical attention (depending on the study) now happen in the unvaccinated. If you've not been vaccinated yet, it's not too late, but remember that it's roughly six weeks from your first shot until you achieve full immunity, and that may be a helluva gauntlet to have to run given what's going on at the moment.

I'm not personally worried about the Delta Variant. I'm fully vaccinated, tend to hang out with people who work in health care or who have careers that depend on COVID risks being reduced, and who therefore lined up for a jab as soon as they were able.

I have a small chance of contracting a breakthrough infection and a very small chance of that infection making me seriously ill. This passes my test of being less risky than getting in a car routinely (1/8400 chance of death this year), so I'm not going to dwell on it. I am slightly concerned about the Delta variant mutating again in an unvaccinated population to become even more virulent, but I'm not going to borrow trouble.

There is good news as well. A study out of Yale that was published today computed that vaccines have so far saved about 300,000 US lives and promise to continue saving many more.

As bad as the pandemic has been on individuals, the health system, the economy, and our collective psyches, it could have been worse.

The original SARS virus (COVID is officially classified as SARS-2) had a mortality rate of 14%. If COVID were similar, we'd have nearly five million US citizens dead over the last 15 months (about one person in 75). Maybe the next pandemic will bring us that.

There will be another one. Hopefully, not for some years. But they come 'round regular as the seasons. All we can do is try to prepare in advance and hope our leaders don't take a wrecking ball to the public health system just prior to the occurrence.

><del>

I'm having new headshots taken this weekend. The last professional ones I had done are now more than 15 years old. (I must admit

I no longer look like I did in my early 40s.) I just got my hair cut short for summer which I hope will make me look distinguished rather than dorky.

I'm itching to get back on stage in something.

There usually isn't a lot of theater around here in the late summer/fall because—football, so I'm holding out hope of booking something challenging for the holidays or early in the new year. There are a few projects coming up that I'm interested in. We'll see what happens.

⚓

I'm trying to think of a good story. This one's a short one and goes back to my senior year of high school. I'll leave the names out of it but my high school friends will know who it's about. It comes to mind because—theater.

When I was in high school, our campus went through a significant expansion plan building several new buildings at once. One of these was an arts center to create new studio space for visual art and a new theater space. Prior to this, the theater program had used the chapel—which had, for instance, no way to access the stage right wings without climbing a ladder through a window.

Teenage me wandered into the new building for the first time, walked onto the stage, looked up at the flies, and was smitten. I wanted to know how to use these tools to create art, so I immediately signed up for technical theater and found that my calling was in stage management.

Some months later, I was stage managing a production of that old chestnut, *You Can't Take It With You*. It was mid-December. We were rehearsing up through the break, then coming back to tech and perform in January.

The cast and crew were mainly overachievers of one kind or another. The guy playing Mr. DePinna found out on the day of one of our last rehearsals before the holiday break that he'd been accepted to

Harvard on their early decision program. In celebration, his parents gave him a bottle of champagne which he brought to rehearsal. Everyone had a swallow in a Dixie cup to toast his good fortune.

The next day the whole cast and crew were called into the principal's office. We were all to be suspended for drinking on campus. Pandemonium.

We all went home for Christmas vacation two days early. That evening, 20 sets of irate parents descended.

They were reassured that the school realized the offense was somewhat ridiculous and that no names were being taken, no records being kept. But they felt that they had to enforce the rule to keep something more problematic from occurring in the future.

My parents laughed about the whole thing as they knew I was far from a troublemaker, besides which they'd allowed us kids small amounts of alcohol at family celebrations for years and knew that a sip of champagne wasn't anything to me.

This was the only "serious" trouble I ever got into during my high school years.

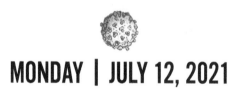

MONDAY | JULY 12, 2021

RIGHT ON SCHEDULE and completely unsurprisingly, the Delta variant of COVID is starting to spike in red states.

There are now more cases of COVID in Arkansas than there were in July of 2020. New hot spots are emerging in Nevada, Louisiana, and Florida. The curve is shifting upward again at a steep pace.

The relative numbers of cases remain low, but it's not going to stay that way with a more infectious strain and large unvaccinated populations in which it can easily run rampant.

The number of deaths daily is back up in the 100s nationally, not on the scale of 2-3000 a day at the peak of the winter surge, but definitely going the wrong direction, especially as the individuals now heading to intensive care units (and, for too many, ultimately the morgue) are tending to be in the 20-60 age group. Older folk have, for the most part, gotten their vaccines and are less likely to congregate in groups.

It's become clear from the data that we have separated into two distinct populations when it comes to public health, divided by politics into red and blue for want of a better shorthand. Blue populations are much more likely to be vaccinated, and in regions where they are dominant, the line against COVID is holding. Red populations are less likely to be vaccinated and are playing host to the vast majority (upwards of 95%) of new infections.

Data out of Florida shows that case rates in red voting counties are double those in blue voting counties. We here in Alabama, currently in last place when it comes to the percentage of the adult population who are fully vaccinated (not yet to 40%), can't seem to get anyone out to vaccine centers so they have, for the most part, shut down. There is plenty of vaccine to be had through commercial pharmacies and county health departments, but few takers.

I'm waiting for Delta to fully take hold. It's here. It will happen. We could easily see local numbers similar to last year.

I don't know what to do about it. I think there's little I can do as an individual other than to offer gentle encouragement on a one-to-one basis with patients and their families. (Almost all of my friends and acquaintances are vaccinated.)

I will also answer questions and try to dispel myths. But when a political party at its rallies and conventions has turned anti-vaccine rhetoric into applause lines, there's not much else to do but hunker down and let them learn the hard way. If I were running a political party, I would not want to take positions that were likely to kill off my most ardent adherents. But that's just me.

What happens when numbers really start to take off in August? I don't know, but I plan on continuing to observe and write and help us all muddle through this rather peculiar time in history.

Will the completely different political realities of blue and red America devolve into civil war?

I certainly hope not, but I put nothing past the major mental health crisis the country seems to be going through. But I think an actual shooting war would be difficult as the populations are so inter-mixed.

There are blue and red states, but even in the red states, the cities and economic engines are blue. It would be very bad for business to round up all your educated city dwellers and run them out of town. The Khmer Rouge tried this in the 1970s, and we all know how well that turned out.

Perhaps we will go the way of 1980s Northern Ireland with blue and red neighborhoods and a sort of no man's land in between. I don't think either side would stand for that as waste ground and barbed wire in the middle of subdivisions is bad for property values and like-ly against HOA policies.

I think we're going to be stuck in a sort of mutual revulsion for a while longer until some sort of major existential threat forces us back together again. One would think a global pandemic would have done it, but obviously, that's not the case.

Today was definitely a Monday at work.

No COVID, but a lot of significant mental health issues com-plicating family dynamics and patient care. Individuals have just reached their breaking point due to societal stress. Brains are awash in catecholamines. When you add eldercare responsibilities on top of all that, things are starting to go a bit haywire.

The current elder generation, with their very long lives, doesn't die rapidly. They decline slowly over years to decades. Children who take them in, thinking it's going to be a year or two, are feeling run-down after a decade or more with no end in sight. COVID has made communal living for the elderly a less attractive option, and hiring in-home care, not a Medicare benefit, is prohibitively expensive for most.

It's going to get even worse over the next decade when you add in the denial of the realities of aging evidenced by the mindset of the Baby Boom. Marching into the future, if I have day-after-workday-after-workday like today, I won't be able to stick with it for long.

I can absorb a lot with my empathic abilities but I have my limits. My usual ten-hour workday stretched to twelve today, and I arrived home with no energy to do much of anything other than feed the cats. The legal cases I am working on will have to wait.

I no longer think I have to end these posts with my litany of wash your hands, wear your mask, stay distant. Only the first of these is really required if you're fully vaccinated and moving among other vaccinated populations. That, however, may change as the variant spreads.

There are more and more reported breakthrough cases of COVID infection in the fully vaccinated including some clusters. However, the vast majority of infections are not life-threatening and can be treated at home.

Just use common sense out there. And if you have unvaccinated friends or family, gently urge them to begin the process now before things start to get hairy later this summer.

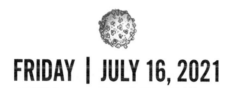

FRIDAY | JULY 16, 2021

T HE NEWS FROM COVIDLAND IS BLEAK.

The numbers are trending up at rates not seen since the major surge last fall. The Ozarks are the canary in the coal mine, likely due to Memorial Day revelry in Branson, Missouri and environs. Now, six or seven weeks later, the hospitals there are full, the death rates are spiking, and they are as overwhelmed as they were six or eight months ago.

But there's a difference this time around.

Last year, there was a feeling of camaraderie and cooperation in health care. Everyone was running on adrenaline and a sense of mission and purpose. Then, this spring, through the miracle of vaccination, numbers came down, the pressure came off, and exhausted healthcare workers took stock.

Some retired, some transferred to less stressful jobs, but the feeling was that the war, if not won, had at least moved into mop-up operations. Then, anti-vaccine frenzy took hold, and now, here we are.

We're no longer running a race against time with a swiftly moving pandemic that's gobsmacked us all upside the head. We're now dealing with a totally preventable disease process that would be well on its way to control, at least on the domestic front, had not a deliberate campaign of disinformation interrupted the flow of vaccine to the population, causing many states to end up with less than half of their healthy adults protected.

Add to this a faster spreading Delta variant, and we're all off to the races again. Only this time, those falling ill are younger and have made a deliberate choice to set themselves up for infection. Meanwhile, an exhausted healthcare system is running out of empathy.

I am not, at heart, a conspiracy theorist. I know far too much about group dynamics to believe that evil cabals can secretly manipulate the world undetected.

However, there must be some sort of strategic reason that explains why one of the two major political parties seems to be willing to tolerate the willful flaunting of the most basic public health precepts.

All I can come up with is that a good deal of the current administration's credibility rests on its proven ability to move rapidly to bring the pandemic under control. Therefore, if the pandemic surges again, with a little help from political rhetoric flouting the rather miraculous reduction of infection through vaccination, the end result serves to undercut the administration in power.

I hate to think that one party is willing to sacrifice lives as so much collateral damage to one-up the other party. I view that as ethically reprehensible. But our politics have become so screwy. I wouldn't put it past the backroom deal makers.

Locally, numbers are up about 50% over last week. Positivity rates of testing are surging. A number of acquaintances of my generation have fallen seriously ill despite being vaccinated. No one has died in that group yet but I know it's coming eventually.

Life here goes on relatively normally.

I'm not worried about myself, but I am wondering what we're going to have to do to keep us from going back to last winter. Full lockdowns are politically unpalatable. Do we go back to full mask mandate/social distancing rules? If the vaccines become fully approved, which is likely to happen within a month or two, do we start mandating them? Do we require vaccine passports for entry into public space?

There are no easy answers.

I'm being judicious with mask use, keeping my hands washed,

and staying somewhat distanced from populations of mixed vaccine status. What else can I do?

I went out on a limb last night.

I was invited to be a storyteller at an event to benefit a local library system. It was a spoken word night with half a dozen storytellers and a few poets.

I arrived, looked at the line-up, and my heart sank.

I recognized more than a few names as folk with significant spoken word cred—the kind I've heard on NPR and at poetry readings around town.

What in the heck was I doing in this group?

I've never been asked to do something like this before. I had rehearsed a couple of possible stories in my head but really had no idea what I was going to do. Fortunately, my slot was somewhat late on the bill. I had a chance to listen to some masters go first. That helped me get a sense of what was playing well to the audience.

When it was my turn, I headed up front, grabbed the mic, thought to myself, "Well, here goes nothing," and entered the zone I go into when I do a public speech or am interviewed on television.

It's hard to explain, but my usual brain gets tucked away in a little corner of my head and a whole different piece of my brain comes out and takes over; I just go along for the ride. I don't know where it comes from or how it operates, but this piece of me is assured, rarely nervous, well-spoken, and pretty nimble.

Ten minutes later, I was done. Then I fell apart inside and questioned every choice I'd made and word I'd spoken.

I've never really been able to do stand-up. I admire those who can because of the difficulty of balancing the humor, the audience expectation, and the need to be true to your material. I don't get stage fright easily but I think I would in a comedy club.

Tommy used to accuse me of always seeking a spotlight. I don't think that's true. I think when I let that piece of me come out (and I have to name him something; I just don't know what), he just knows how to communicate and the spotlight finds him.

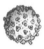

TUESDAY | JULY 20, 2021

ASTEN YOUR SEATBELTS, it's going to be a bumpy night."

So goes the famous line. I have a feeling the bumps are going to be lasting a lot longer than tonight, this week, or next month.

Humans changed their behavior again and the virus has been doing quietly what the virus does in the shadows the last few weeks. We're all waking up to the fact that it's everywhere again.

You all remember the pattern from last year: behavior change leads to a rise in cases in two to three weeks and a spike in death rates two to three weeks after that.

Two weeks ago was a holiday weekend. Lots of opportunities for humans to gather, so they did. Cases were relatively low. The Delta Variant was out there but rare. But with its increased transmissibility, it took advantage of closer human contact to spread. Exponential math took over from there.

The Delta Variant is now 83% of total COVID cases in the US.

Case numbers are rising in every state. The absolute numbers are still below where we were six or seven months ago, but all the trends are wrong.

Case positivity is back over 5% but a lot of testing sites have shut down so we don't know if we're getting an accurate read or not. State health departments are all over the map in getting their data to federal sources. It's hard to know what's going on in real-time, but we're back to adding nearly 100,000 cases a week.

The death toll continues to mount slowly. We'll have no problem surpassing the Civil War casualty figures in a couple of months at this rate. And half the adult population is either unvaccinated or under-vaccinated—nearly three-quarters of the adult population here in Alabama.

It's not like it's hard to find a vaccine these days.

The times of searching online every night and driving four counties over are long gone. Vials are going begging for willing arms. And it's not like they haven't been tried out in hundreds of millions of people.

They may still be under emergency use authorization and "experimental" but the safety record has been excellent, data is being submitted to the FDA, and they are likely to receive full formal approval shortly.

I am beginning to lose my patience with those who are foregoing vaccines for political reasons or obviously disprovable misinformation. The message I am getting is that you have a fundamental lack of respect for others in society, most particularly those who go out on a limb routinely to see to your health and safety. Doctors, nurses, and other caregivers are exhausted after this past year and a half and they're gearing up to go back into hell again.

A friend was involved in a traffic accident today. He went to the UAB emergency room and was practically chased out as the whole place was swamped with new-onset COVID patients. It's no wonder every doctor and nurse and therapist in my age group that I speak to is considering their exit strategy and retirement. No human should be asked to bear this, especially when it's completely unnecessary.

Rant over.

Well, maybe not.

I'm going to be on more than just a rant if I have to cancel my vacation plans again this year due to virus resurgence and a need to lock down and work toward flattening curves again. (Grump. Grump.)

I'm also trying to figure out what to do about masking in the face of the rise of Delta. (Doesn't that sound like a really bad action movie with Jean-Claude Van Damme?)

I mask at work when in clinical space as do all employees and patients. We may be around people who cannot be vaccinated for various medical reasons or whose immune systems cannot mount proper responses.

I don't mask when gathered with a small group of vaccinated friends. I don't mask outdoors. Where I am stuck is going into stores or other places where the general public gathers.

Masking isn't so much about protecting yourself. It's about protecting others. (People forget this.) It works and works well when it is universal. But if you're the only person wearing one, it's not so protective.

With no further mandates in place, few are wearing masks locally. Do I slip one on when heading into the Piggly Wiggly (I don't mind), or do I just trust in my vaccinated status and my relatively good health to keep me from becoming too ill, and then isolate should I become symptomatic?

I've taken to writing out my frustrations here.

Others in my family are more visually inclined and create art. My sister, who has always been the artistic one, has made quite a career as an illustrator over the years, currently working predominantly in ink on human skin. (I'm referring to tattooing, not to some weird Ed

Gein thing.) She did the cover art for Volume One of *The Accidental Plague Diaries* and has promised a suitable encore for Volume Two.

My father is a decent watercolorist. He's also very clever with his hands. He made many of our toys growing up. My nieces are both quite talented at drawing and graphic arts. My aunt became quite well known in the refined world of handmade papers and books after exploring Japanese woodblock techniques.

The visual gene skipped me. When I pick up paint or colored pencils, the results tend to look like something a kindergartener left on the refrigerator.

Tommy and Steve got the gay visual gene. They were both the kind of guys you could give some construction paper, a glue gun, and some crèpe streamers to and they'd emerge from the garage with a parade float after an hour. Not me. I did get the show tune gene and the brunch-with-too-many-mimosas gene, though.

>——<

I tried my hand at visual arts once.

In high school, we were required to have a year of visual arts to graduate. I took graphic arts my junior year. It encompassed basic drawing techniques, watercolor, various mixed media things, block-printing, and the only thing that I was any good at—batik. (I still have a couple of my high school batik pieces hanging around.)

Our teacher was a wonderfully laid-back guy with a droll sense of humor who was actually interested in what was going on in our adolescent heads. Teaching art was only one of his careers.

On weekends, he was the minister for a Unitarian Universalist congregation in one of Seattle's suburbs. He was my first introduction to UU (although he didn't push it onto impressionable minds). I was raised Congregationalist, the most liberal of the Protestant Mainline denominations, so UU wasn't that far off from what I came from.

I don't think he thought much of my potential artistic talents (or

240

lack thereof) although he was complimentary of my imagination and my liking to twist assignments in some interesting way. We got along quite well.

I didn't think that much about him or what he taught me for years after high school until a simple essay he wrote in his church job caught on in the 1990s and, all of a sudden there was a poster on everyone's wall. The essay was entitled All I Needed to Know I Learned in Kindergarten, and Robert Fulghum, my high school art teacher, became an international name.

There's a quote from that famous essay that I think we all need to remember at this moment in history while we forge our way ahead.

Share everything.

Play fair.

Don't hit people.

Put things back where you found them.

Clean up your own mess.

Don't take things that aren't yours.

Say you're sorry when you hurt somebody.

Wash your hands before you eat.

SUNDAY | JULY 25, 2021

KEEP HOPING that I'm going to run out of things to write about COVID, but this hasn't happened yet.

If the population of the US will start behaving rationally and doing a few basic common sense things, I might. I am, however, not overly hopeful.

The poison of misinformation has permeated the body politic too deeply to be gotten rid of easily. The end result is now 611,000 dead Americans with the numbers steadily climbing again.

In the last day or so, I have seen news reports from the UK on an anti-mask/anti-vaccine/anti-everything rally where one of the speakers was calling for the execution of physicians and nurses for advocating public health measures.

Another one from Israel on an anti-vaccine crowd laying siege to the new prime minister's home.

And yet another from Brazil where the president was threatening a military coup to keep his beliefs about the "harmlessness" of COVID firmly in place.

It's all a wakeup call to remind me that the pandemic is not a domestic, but a global problem, and that the reactionary forces I see locally are not limited to red states.

Any place that allows the coronavirus to spread unchecked is going to serve as a reservoir for additional mutations and reinfections into the population as a whole.

The vaccines seem to be holding the line. There are studies suggesting that they are not necessarily fully effective at keeping a vaccinated person from contracting a Delta infection, but the data available suggests that a vaccinated person will not progress to the frightening complications that lead to hospitalization and death. Those, at this point, seem to be limited to the unvaccinated among us.

The few vaccinated who have succumbed to Delta infection all seem to have had serious underlying illnesses of various stripes. There have been almost no cases of healthy vaccinated people catching Delta and then becoming critically ill. I'm waiting for the data to come in as to whether a booster shot will be helpful. If it is suggested, I'll be among the first in line.

242

I went to a fundraiser for a local theater company last night. Drinks, edible tidbits, some singing, and an art auction. I bought a lovely metal piece which will go on one of my terrace walls.

The theater folk of Birmingham, starved for gatherings of this type, turned out en masse and several hundred folk were there. I wore a mask when not eating and drinking through most of the evening.

I trust that most of the people there use good judgment, but if we continue to mask indoors in crowded situations, even for a little while, we'll be able to help break transmission chains while the authorities start figuring out the messaging necessary to get vaccination rates up.

It's been very interesting to see what's happening in Republican political circles over the last two weeks. During the spring when vaccinations were quickly reaching arms and case rates began to plummet, it became fashionable for them to decry public health measures as an overreaction or an unnecessary burden on people.

These ideas, amplified through their media machine, became loud enough and widespread enough to more or less level off the vaccination rates nationally over the last month, coinciding with the rise of Delta. That's why we're in the current fix we're in.

As it has become increasingly clear that this attitude is directly harming the Republican base, a certain amount of internecine warfare has broken out in the party between Republicans who understand that there's a time when political rhetoric is destructive and Republicans who have lost the ability to stand for anything and can only stand against the prevailing attitudes of the day.

I'm wondering what happens when the Republican base starts to figure out that they were put in harm's way and allowed to sicken and die as so much collateral damage to allow their leaders to deny the Democratic administration "a win" on vaccine delivery and ending the pandemic?

This afternoon I have a Spolin improvisation class with some of my favorite theater buddies. It's a small group of people who know that vaccines are their way back to doing what they love so I won't mask for that.

I'm trying to use good judgment without going overboard. I wash my hands, don't squeeze up on other people if I don't need to, I wear my mask where warranted, and I have my shots.

This is what we can all do as individuals for the good of society at present.

WEDNESDAY | JULY 28, 2021

COVID'S BUSTIN' OUT ALL OVER. All over the ICU and morgue. I wish I didn't have to say that, but the numbers are soaring locally with Alabama having gone from a couple of hundred daily diagnoses at the beginning of the month, to about 1,000 cases a day mid-month, to about 2,000 cases a day at the end of last week, to nearly 3,000 cases a day this week. It's the power of exponential numbers manifesting in real time.

We're back over 1,000 hospitalized patients statewide, a place we haven't been since February, just as the vaccinations were really beginning to gear up. Things show no signs of letting up.

I haven't seen the numbers for UAB yet, but all the pieces are moving to get the hospital ready for full-scale inundation. Elective procedures are beginning to be postponed. Drive-thru testing sites are being ramped back up. Medical services are limiting transfers in.

We remain behind the curve as the Delta variant didn't really start spreading in Alabama until this month. Given the well-known delays between diagnoses, hospitalization rates, and death rates, we won't start to see a major crush on the hospitals for another week or two. Death rates will start going up beginning mid-August.

To see where we're going just look at the Ozark area of Southern Missouri and Northern Arkansas. Delta arrived early via Memorial Day Weekend in Branson. Now, eight weeks later, every hospital in the region is full. I have seen reports from physicians in the area that there are no ICU beds to be had in any of the surrounding states for desperately ill people, and that they are significantly short-staffed.

The current surge is very different from the surges of 2020. Those were based in dense urban environments with large numbers of international travelers—New York, San Francisco, Los Angeles, Seattle. The current surge is hitting small towns and rural areas where the infrastructure is nowhere near as robust.

When the numbers really begin to increase in Alabama next month, UAB and Birmingham will be OK. We have a strong medical infrastructure with a number of excellent hospitals. Rural Alabama, with its healthcare systems already weakened to the point of collapse by the political refusal of successive Republican administrations to take the Medicaid expansion, will not fare so well.

I'm not sure that the smaller hospitals that serve a huge portion of the population are going to be able to survive the coming crisis. When they shut their doors due to lack of funds, lack of staff, and a crush of patients they are ill-equipped to handle, what comes next? When every ICU bed for a hundred miles is occupied by a COVID patient on a ventilator, what happens to the usual parade of heart attacks, strokes, traffic accidents, gunshot victims, and all of the other things that arrive seeking acute care on a daily basis?

This is what infuriates me about the political push to undermine vaccines which has been conducted through certain media outlets since the change in administration. It's not just about you and your personal choice. It's about a healthcare system that was just beginning to recover from crisis and is now slipping back into it.

It's about callous disregard for the toll that a preventable illness is going to exact not just on you but on the people who care for you, physically and emotionally. It's about the denial of a more open life to the part of society that stepped up, washed their hands, masked up, socially distanced, and got their vaccines—all tried and true public health measures—and whose hard work is being undone by people who somehow believe that viral illness works along partisan lines.

Given the infectiousness of the Delta variant and the way exponential math works, it's entirely possible that the vast majority of the 100 million or so American adults without vaccines will be exposed to it in the next two or three months. That's another 500,000-1,500,000 unnecessary deaths that could be coming by the end of the year.

〜

I'm tired of writing about COVID. I really am.

It's been over 16 months now since the first entry in what has become two volumes now of *The Accidental Plague Diaries*. I would love to write more about theater and travel and interesting people and reminiscences and art, but every time I think I'm out, I get pulled back in again by a story that, as of yet, has no end. It seems to have become my place in life to chronicle all of this so that I and those of you who didn't give up three paragraphs ago can continue to process the ongoing saga.

So I continue to write.

In the meantime, back to the litany. Wash your hands. Wear your mask indoors around people you don't know. Social distance when you can. UAB is going back to indoor masking in all buildings unless you're in your own office.

Get your vaccine. It's not too late. A pharmacist friend told me that community demand is going back up (three vaccines a day last week; 20 vaccines a day this week), but there's still plenty to be had.

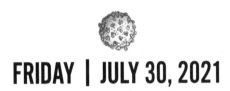

FRIDAY | JULY 30, 2021

THERE'S ANOTHER THUNDERSTORM rolling into town. Lightning on the horizon is flashing through my bedroom window. It seems apropos at the start of a weekend which is likely to be defined as the one in which the state of Alabama finally woke up to the realities of the Delta variant.

Those of us who've been paying attention for the last month have been watching the numbers and trends with some alarm, but the general population has been blithely conducting its business in a serene optimism that pandemic dangers have passed. Over the last few days, the news has become too major to ignore. In both public and private spheres, folk have woken up to the fact that we're in for a wild ride.

What's happened?

The rolling seven-day average of COVID cases in Alabama, which was about 200 a day at the first of the month, is now ten times that with a positivity rate pushing 20%. The number of hospitalized in Alabama is also up tenfold over the course of the month with more rolling in every hour. The rate of new diagnoses is shooting up in a steeper curve than even during the worst of this past winter's surge.

Delta isn't playing around.

Its R0 (the number of people a carrier is able to infect) is much higher than the original strains of COVID. Where that was between

2 and 3, Delta is somewhere between 5 and 10. That doesn't seem like much difference until you realize we're dealing with exponential math. A disease with an R0 of 2.5 will spread to about 100 people after six iterations. A disease with an R0 of 7.5 will spread to nearly 25,000 people in the same six iterations.

There are hysterical headlines appearing regularly: "Vaccines not as Effective as Thought'; "Vaccinated can Spread the Virus as Easily as the Unvaccinated." When you look closely at this material, much of which is from non-journalistic and non-science sources, you find that much of what is written is misrepresenting the actual data on which the sensationalism is based, so I'm going to try and take a minute to parse out what we really know about the Delta variant at this time.

Mind you, much of what we know is somewhat sketchy as it's not been around that long. Some of this comes from studies done in India, where the mutation that caused the variant originally arose. Some of this comes from studies done in the UK which had the Delta variant earlier than most Western countries due to its cultural/travel links with India.

Some of this comes from a study of a cluster outbreak of the Delta variant stemming from the traditional gathering of gay men in Provincetown, Massachusetts over the 4th of July weekend which led to a significant spreading among a crowd of healthy and fully vaccinated folk who likely spent a good deal of their time on the dance floor.

The Delta variant is not a new disease. It is a mutation of the coronavirus which changes COVID into a form that is more easily transmissible. There is some evidence that it may also be more virulent and cause worse disease.

The vaccines administered so far have been effective. But they are not 100% effective against a breakthrough infection. Somewhere around 10% of vaccinated people can develop the disease if exposed.

However, vaccinated people have had much milder diseases. In the Provincetown cluster mentioned above, more than 1,000 cases were identified. Fewer than 20 required hospitalization (usually short-term) and no one to date has died.

We don't know if a third booster vaccine will improve immunity against Delta. There are no recommendations for this, and the federal system which pays for vaccines will not authorize administration of a third vaccine at this time. The original cohort of people who volunteered to be guinea pigs for the vaccine a year ago are being studied and we may know more about this from their data in a few months.

It appears that some (but not all) people with breakthrough infections can transmit the virus to others. For this reason, the CDC is again recommending indoor masking for the vaccinated. This is a new finding which is why the CDC is changing its advice.

Science constantly updates itself with new empirical evidence. When the CDC changes guidelines, it's not because it's being inconsistent, it's because it's learning new things about the virus and is trying to help us adapt.

Unvaccinated people are highly vulnerable to the Delta variant. It takes roughly 6-8 weeks from initiation of vaccination to achieve full vaccination status with Pfizer or Moderna, so the time to get vaccinated is now, not next week. Hospitalization rates are skyrocketing due to the large percentages of unvaccinated—and, therefore, vulnerable people—and the infectiousness of Delta.

The best weapons we have against Delta are the ones we have always had. Wash your hands. Keep your distance when you can. Mask up (again) when indoors with those you don't know. It's a piece of cloth, not barbed wire or chainmail. Masks work, but only when we all wear them.

I don't think we need to go into lockdown. The vaccines are effective, and the majority of those most vulnerable to the virus have been vaccinated. We just need to exercise common sense.

Those who have regular contact with vulnerable adults such as those working in health care need to be vaccinated if they have not been already. It's not about you, it's about the people you care for. Vaccine mandates are coming and will increase once the FDA moves vaccines from emergency use to approved status.

Studies of the vaccination of children under 12 are ongoing. We may have results in a few months but not before the start of the school year. Universal masking in schools is a good idea, no matter what your political leanings.

While there are lots of news stories about children's hospitals filling up, children, as a whole, do not remain at major risk of serious disease. If you have children too young for vaccination, the best thing to do to protect them is to ensure that all family members and close contacts 12 and over are vaccinated.

It remains to be seen what's going to happen to the mortality statistics. The health system has gotten much better at treating the disease than it was a year and a half ago, and the people succumbing currently, in the unvaccinated population, tend to be younger and physiologically healthier.

The mortality rate may not skyrocket the way the case rate is currently doing but we're going to have to wait a few weeks to find out. I don't wish ill on anyone but I also don't understand those who have refused to take a few simple steps to protect themselves from a deadly disease.

My favorite story about exponential math is one I remember from an elementary school textbook, one I likely had in fifth or sixth grade. In it, they described a legend connected with the invention of chess.

Apparently, the Sultan of some unnamed kingdom was so impressed with the game that he invited the inventor to his palace and asked him what he would like as a reward. The inventor replied that he asked for very little, just some grains of rice. One grain for the first square, two grains for the second square, four grains for the third square, eight grains for the fourth square, and so on, doubling with each square.

The Sultan took the inventor for a fool, cried "Done!" and asked for a bag of rice to be brought. The Sultan, of course, made the mistake of thinking that exponential math works like linear math when it does not. There are 64 squares on a chessboard. Two to the 64th power is somewhere in the quintillions and would generate enough rice to bury the entire state of California to a depth of five feet.

There aren't that many people in the state of Alabama so, if the disease is that contagious, it will spread very, very rapidly through the susceptible population and likely burn itself out relatively quickly. This is more or less what happened in India. I just hope it manages to do so without crushing the health system and with a minimum of mortality and severe morbidity, but we shall see what we shall see.

In the meantime, you all know the drill. Get those masks back out and put them on indoors in public. Keep your distance. Wash your hands. Convince your loved ones to go get a vaccine NOW.

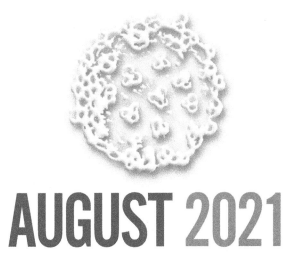

AUGUST 2021

Too Darn Hot

SUNDAY | AUGUST 1, 2021

S TEVE DIED 20 YEARS AGO TODAY.

It was an ordinary day, like so many of the days before. His lung disease had been a bit worse over the past week with some drop in his oxygen saturation making him more confused, but we were over the worst of that and he was coming back to his usual baseline orneriness.

Tameka, his caretaker when I was at work, came at her usual time. She and I exchanged pleasantries while I finished my coffee and headed out the door. Steve was at his art table at the dining room window, working on a watercolor with a pen and ink overlay of some flowers.

The weather was sunny and he had a couple of visitors lined up for the morning. His hospice chaplain was due to stop by, as was another friend, to shoot the breeze for a while before lunch and then, if he felt up to it, an outing with Tameka to just get out of the house. The two of them were quite the pair, rodding around town in his blue Mustang convertible.

At about 11:30 that morning, after enjoying his visitors, he was resting on the couch in the living room. He stood up, turned to Tameka, said "I don't feel so good," and then dropped like a rock to the floor. His heart, which had been under incredible strain trying to pump blood through his increasingly fibrotic lungs, simply gave up and stopped. He was dead pretty much as soon as he went down.

Tameka called me in a panic. It was a Wednesday and I was on VA duty doing house calls for their home-based primary care program. In those days, we piled the whole team into a van and did home invasion of all the disciplines at once. With Steve being so ill, I knew I might have to race back at any time, so I had taken to following the van in my own car.

I told Tameka to relax, call the hospice, and I would get home as soon as I could. I excused myself from the home visit, got in my car, and started to race across town. The phone rang again. It was the police who had somehow been summoned and gotten there before the hospice nurse, informing me that Steve was most definitely dead.

I don't remember much after that point.

I know I got home.

Steve was lying on the floor where he had fallen and was most definitely no longer among the living. I calmed Tameka down and sent her home. The hospice nurse showed up as did the funeral home transport. I kissed him goodbye on the forehead and made sure that Patrick, his cat, was able to sniff and recognize that he was gone.

A few friends showed up. I needed to keep myself busy so I kept doing stupid things like unloading his pillboxes just to keep my hands and brain doing something other than thinking about what had just happened. I called our pastor, who was out of state awaiting the birth of her first grandchild. I decided on having the memorial quickly that coming Sunday afternoon.

What I remember most was just feeling.

I've never been good at emotions or understanding them. To this day, I cannot always tell when an emotional response is positive or negative, much less what the emotion actually is. It's odd. I'm very good at understanding and identifying emotions in others but not so good at doing it within my own brain. Even a few courses of psychotherapy have not been able to help me much with this one.

I suppose that day it was truly a mixture of many things, both positive and negative.

Love for Steve.

I was 39. We had been together since I was 26. He had been my constant companion through my mature adulthood up to that point.

Loss and regret.

We had no more time together to build new memories. Relief that his suffering (and by extension, mine) was over. Fear at what would come next. I had no idea how to be alone as a functioning adult.

At that time, I also had no idea that Tommy was out there. We had met each other when he had waited on me and Steve at the local Olive Garden, but I have no recollection of this.

I had not yet been prodded back into the world of performance, music, and theater. I was thinking it might be time to return to the West Coast somewhere.

>———◦

613,000 plus American families have gone through that shock and loss over the last 18 months.

The current death toll from COVID is inching up but isn't accelerating at the rate it once did. This may not hold true much longer.

Both Louisiana and Florida are reporting numbers of new cases on a par with last winter at the worst of that surge. Other under-vaccinated states are starting to accelerate in the same way. It will be a month before we know what that's going to do to the death toll.

I spent my last post trying to lay out the facts about what's happening to us with the spread of the Delta variant which is significantly more transmissible than the Alpha variant which caused last winter's surge. I'm not sure what I can add to that.

Breakthrough infections in the vaccinated are definitely increasing. Fortunately, the vaccine is doing its job and the majority remain relatively mild. The chance of a vaccinated person dying from COVID is somewhere between 1/100,000 and 1/1,000,000 which is roughly the same as being struck by lightning in any given year (1/500,000).

If you're vaccinated, don't panic. You're protected.

The new recommendation to mask up again isn't so much about you as it is about the protection of society and the unvaccinated, especially kids. Masks are more about protecting others than they are about protecting you; they are a mark of social altruism. It comes from the recent data out of Provincetown around the Fourth of July weekend which showed that fully vaccinated people are capable of spreading Delta, even if they aren't getting that sick themselves.

The Provincetown data are very good. The CDC has gone on record as to how well people cooperated and helped them trace contacts. They were able to map out infections with accuracy and ease that they weren't used to seeing.

That's because we're dealing with gay men here. This isn't their first time at the pandemic rodeo. They know what to do and how to be good citizens, even though their country isn't always great at repaying them.

Now, as gay men, when they gather en masse, tend to crowd themselves into bars and onto dance floors, there may have been a bit more ease of transmission going on than you will find at your neighborhood Publix—unless you're living in West Hollywood.

I've been getting a lot of questions about kids. I'm not a pediatrician or an elementary educator (except for Sunday school), but I do try to keep up on the latest. The political forces that are trying to ban masking in schools are crazy, but laws have been passed.

Very young children before school age may have issues with masks but once they get to Kindergarten, they'll comply if it's reinforced. And they can take them off outside at recess. Masks will not stunt their growth or lower their oxygen or any of those other things.

There are cultures in which that part of the body is routinely covered and they don't have any issues. We just believe in Western society that if you cover any part of your face, you have something to hide.

At the moment, masking should be universal indoors in schools. The Delta variant appears to hit kids a bit harder than the Alpha variant. There have certainly been more hospitalizations. Whether it has increased mortality for children we don't yet know. Things might change as more and more adults get vaccinated.

Studies are ongoing as to whether it is safe to vaccinate kids. There should be at least some preliminary results this fall. In the meantime, how do you best protect your kids? If they are 12 or older, have them vaccinated. If they are under 12, make sure all of the adults around them are vaccinated and that they mask up when indoors at school or in other public places.

So what to do? Repeat after me.

Wear your mask indoors in public (unless actively eating or drinking). Wash your hands. Keep a reasonable distance from those you don't know. Get your shots.

There's no need to go back into lockdown if we just do a few simple things for our friends and neighbors.

WEDNESDAY | AUGUST 4, 2021

WELL, WHERE ARE WE?

A quick summation of some recent news stories: Louisiana's largest hospital is completely out of beds. The number of people hospitalized with COVID in Florida is roughly the same as it was back at the peak of this past winter's surge.

The total number of cases diagnosed in the US so far is something over 35 million (or roughly 10% of the total population) and is going up currently by 100,000 a day. Closer to home, the number of hospitalizations in Alabama has doubled from two weeks ago, but there's an odd geographic predilection.

The huge increases are in the Gulf Coast and Mobile Bay areas, and not so much in the cities further inland. I put that down to cavorting at the beach over the Fourth of July Weekend and geographic proximity to Louisiana. It's coming our way. Druid City Hospital in Tuscaloosa which was down to seven COVID patients at the first of July now has over 100.

The good news among all these bleak statistics is that if you are fully vaccinated, you need not worry too much. Of the hospitalizations in Alabama between January and July with COVID, 99% were in unvaccinated individuals. Those with breakthrough cases generally recover at home without much incident.

I am adhering to indoor masking recommendations personally. I'm not afraid for myself, but I care enough about my fellow citizens to try and keep from being infected by an asymptomatic carrier. Besides, I have quite the collection of high-fashion masks these days and I go to great pains to match them with my shirt of the day. I also try to get my socks to match but that's sometimes a more difficult task.

><@

The big debate going on at the moment, as we are approaching the first day of school, is school policies regarding masking, social distancing, and safety in the classroom. The Delta variant appears to be somewhat more infectious in children than the Alpha variant of last year. I don't have hard numbers on this but it's alluded to by several trusted sources.

No one wants to go back to virtual school as it wasn't terribly good for either kids or education, so the consensus is that schools will open on their usual schedule. The state of Alabama, kowtowing to political pressure from the right wing of the Republican party, has passed legislation forbidding any use of "vaccine passports", whatever that's supposed to mean (although the legislation has no penalties attached for violations).

The governor has made it quite clear that she will not impose any sort of state mask mandate. At least she hasn't expressly forbidden the use of masks in schools like Florida, Texas, and Arkansas have (where the governor is very sorry he signed the legislation). She's simply kicked the can down to local governance and school boards.

Locally, city schools have announced a mask mandate. The wealthy suburbs are being torn by competing groups of vocal parents—those calling for a mask mandate to protect their kids and those calling for no mask mandates to encourage their kids to have some normalcy in childhood.

I have a couple of thoughts about this.

First, kids are infinitely adaptable. They'll do whatever the culture tells them is proper in regards to dress and behavior. Tell them they have to wear masks, and they will; it's what happens in all those cultures where face veiling is considered a proper standard. It won't hurt them in any way. They'll only rebel against masks if they're getting the information from a trusted adult that they should rebel. Masks aren't going to damage them or their educational experience.

Second, if the first job of governance is to protect the citizenry (something that has been in short supply these last few years), the second job is to make sure that the next generation can grow and develop into functional and competent adults. This means adults have to be adult and put the needs of kids before their own wants sometimes.

Kids need to be around their peers and they need to be educated. The steps we take should ensure these things happen. Masks are a very small price to pay for this to happen safely.

People often forget the purpose of the mask. It's not about you. They don't keep you from getting COVID, but if everyone wears them, they prevent COVID from propagating in the group. That's ultimately more important. They need to be universal in areas of high transmission. They can come off again when transmission rates fall.

I don't have children so I don't have a dog in this fight, but if I did, I'd send them to school with masks for use in the building and tell them to take them off and run around and yell, scream, and sing outside at recess.

To date, roughly 500 children have died of COVID in the US. That's not a lot compared to the total of 615,000 or so deaths we've had so far, but every one of those 500 families is broken, some beyond repair, and 500 lives that were full of potential have been snuffed out at a young age.

We'll never know if there was a Gershwin or a Simone Biles among them. With vaccines, we can protect kids, not by vaccinating them directly (yet—but that may change), but by making sure they are surrounded by adults who care enough about them to reduce their chances of exposure by being themselves vaccinated. That's how herd immunity works. The death of any child from now on is one too many. It's not necessary; we have the tools to protect them.

I really don't understand the political calculus of the right-wing at the moment. The noise machine remains firmly anti-vaccination and continues to spew toxic misinformation to its base. I presume this is to be able to point to the Biden administration and say, "See, they failed to protect you from the pandemic—vote for us!" in next year's midterms.

But the cynical calculations that have been made with innocent people's lives, especially those of children and young adults, are unconscionable. It's as if Governors Abbot and DeSantis and their ilk were standing in front of the altar of Moloch, demanding the population push their children into the flames.

In a decade or two, when this is all an unpleasant memory and today's kids are young adults, those 20- and 30-somethings are going to look at their parents and ask "What did you do to keep me safe during the pandemic?" Some very uncomfortable conversations will follow.

It's all so different from when I was in elementary school and we were lined up for polio, MMR, and other vaccines in the auditorium. I don't recall a single one of us having a parent who complained. They were just thankful that the dreaded diseases of their own childhoods had been beaten back.

⚜

My earliest memory is of polio.

I was not quite two but I vividly remember the little girl who lived next door who walked with braces on her legs. She'd had polio several years before. It's almost the only thing I remember from that very young age, so it must have made a huge impression on me.

We lived in a Connecticut suburb at the time (my father was on the faculty at Yale). I don't remember much about it at all, but when Mad Men came out a few years ago with its depiction of suburban New England life in the early 60s, all of a sudden, memories of various conversations my parents had had about their neighbors and acquaintances from that time came rushing back. And I understood their decision to hightail it to the West Coast in the summer of 1964.

The litany continues: mask indoors in public, wash your hands, get your shots, love your children.

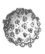

SUNDAY | AUGUST 8, 2021

HOUSTON, WE HAVE A PROBLEM. And Baton Rouge. And Mobile. And Jacksonville. And Little Rock. And, and, and…

The news pouring in from all over on the rise of the Delta variant remains grim. Hospitals and ICUs are full. There are reports of burnt-out healthcare workers simply walking off the job at the end of a shift, unable to stomach more unnecessary death and suffering.

We're back over 100,000 new cases a day across the country. On the first go-round in 2020, it took us nearly eight months to hit that milestone which was reached in the first week of November. It only took about six weeks this time to go from a low of fewer than 7,000 cases a day in early June to where we are now.

A brief reminder on how the virus works.

It has no sentient decision-making capacity. It transfers itself from host to host using to its advantage the behavioral choices of humans to gather in groups. What we are seeing today is the result of our behavioral choices of mid-June when there was a definite feeling that the worst was over and we could start getting back to normal patterns.

What we choose to do today will have no effect on what happens tomorrow. Our behaviors today won't become apparent in the course of the pandemic until mid-to-late September. This lag between behavior and consequence of behavior is a bit of a problem.

Many of us humans don't understand cause and effect. If there isn't a clear temporal association between two things, we have difficulties understanding the relationship. Of course, the opposite is also true. When two things happen in close proximity in time, we want to believe in a relationship even when one does not exist.

Correlation is not causation. I suppose this is, at least in part, one of the reasons why so many of us are susceptible to irrational theories regarding phenomena over scientific fact. The combination of more normal behavioral patterns regarding group activities, relaxing of masking and social distancing standards, and a significant portion of the population rejecting the one thing we have that we know works to keep the virus at bay has led us to our present predicament.

The Delta variant is moving much faster than the previous Alpha variant. It's moving so fast that neither our systems of governance nor our understanding of the patterns of epidemic disease can really keep up with it in real time. The combination of transmissibility and the huge unvaccinated population in the red states is leading to a perfect storm that's going to get a whole lot worse very quickly thanks to the realities of exponential math.

Full hospitals in the cities on the leading edge of this new wave will be replicated elsewhere and the pressures aren't going to let up for some months, even if we decide to lock down again—and I don't see any governmental entity having the stomach to suggest that, especially when the class of individuals with political power is pretty much all vaccinated and relatively protected.

If the numbers go up as rapidly as they could, we're going to see some hospital systems simply unable to cope further—out of beds, out of staff, out of resources. The collateral damage will be everyone else who gets sick from all of the other usual issues that send people off to acute care. They won't have much help. My hospital is gearing up for another time like last winter and is ratcheting down on elective surgeries and other things that might take up hospital beds, saving them for the crunch that has yet to come.

><><

The governors of Texas and Florida continue their contest to see which one can kill a greater percentage of their population. Florida appears to be winning.

Current statistics there show a rate of 132 cases per 100,000 population. If Florida were an independent country, its rate would be the third-highest in the world, behind Martinique and St. Barts. (Those two countries have such small populations that one or two more cases move them up the rankings quite quickly.)

For comparison, Alabama, which is quite high for states, has roughly 50 cases per 100,000 population at the moment. Governor DeSantis, in Florida, to keep the crown, has forbidden school districts from mandating masking on campus or face severe financial penalties. He has also had laws passed forbidding cruise lines from requiring vaccination prior to boarding a cruise ship, perhaps the most perfect environment for viral transmission yet invented. Not to be outdone, Governor Abbott in Texas is busy forbidding contact tracing in public schools and allowing potentially infectious children to attend without a quarantine period.

I'm trying to figure out why elected officials are deliberately doubling down against the advice of every public health and healthcare provider group out there. All I can come up with is that the Republican position on any issue is simply to be against whatever Democrats might be for, and who cares about collateral damage in the form of dead citizens. But then, this is the party that refused to pass common-sense gun legislation after a school full of dead kindergarteners a decade ago. The lives of children don't seem to mean much, likely because they aren't major campaign donors.

The same things are playing out locally, with our own governor refusing to mandate any particular school safety measures and kicking it down to local school districts; things are going about as well as might be expected in this heavily red state.

Roughly 1/3 of Alabama schools will be opening with a mask mandate, 2/3 will not. Locally, the city schools are requiring masks, the county schools are not, and the suburban school districts are all over the map. This is playing out especially contentiously in one of the wealthy suburban school districts where many of the University faculty live and send their kids, and where the school board (three retailers and two attorneys with no education experience among them) have decided that masks are optional but encouraged. This has enraged that portion of the parent base employed in health care. My Facebook feed has been full of screeds against the politics of the moment that would let this happen.

Vaccines continue to hold the line for now. As more and more data comes in, it shows that vaccines aren't the best at preventing infection, which is why we are all aware of a vaccinated person or two with a breakthrough case. Vaccines also aren't the best at preventing someone with a breakthrough infection from being a carrier and spreading it to others. The numbers for both of these things are significantly lower in the vaccinated population but hardly zero.

However, multiple studies from around the world show that vaccinated people are not getting the complications that require hospitalization and aggressive therapy. And the few people who do become that ill while vaccinated are nearly all individuals with serious underlying health concerns independent of COVID. If you're reasonably healthy and vaccinated, your chance of major hospitalization or death is very small. You can, however, still be part of the transmission chain which is why it's important to keep those masks on indoors in public for now.

I spent yesterday at the Magic City Clarinet Festival. The Birmingham Music Club asked me to sponsor it and, as clarinet was my elementary/middle/high school instrument, I was happy to do so. Performances of everything from classical pieces to avant-garde to Dixieland jazz. Masterclasses from professional clarinetists from around the region.

It was well attended for a niche festival, and the venue at the Birmingham Museum of Art, which has great air circulation, was the right place for wind instruments. I dusted off my instrument case, brought it with me, and joined in the grand finale of *Somewhere Over the Rainbow*.

I can still play but it's been a long time since I've played for an audience for anything other than comic effect. The last time the clarinet was out of its case was when I was in *Gypsy*. I dubbed *Clarence and His Clarinet* from the opening scene behind the curtain complete with squeaks. I also played it once in *Politically Incorrect* after a setup where no one in the audience thought I could actually play it.

I started playing in fourth grade. At that time, in the Seattle Public Schools, you were allowed to pick an orchestral instrument and, for a modest fee, the music teacher would teach you to play. My original choice was flute, but after playing around with it for a week, I had a hard time with the embouchure, and couldn't get much sound out of it so I switched to clarinet which I could at least make squawk right away.

Our music teacher was Norma Durst. She played viola in the Seattle Symphony and was an institution, having joined the group in her 20s and playing with them until fading eyesight forced her to retire in her 80s. When she taught me the rudiments of clarinet, she was probably about 50 and in her prime. And she actually had us formed into a school orchestra after only six months or so. Eat your heart out Harold Hill.

It's time for the litany. You should all know it by heart. Wash your hands. Get your shot. Keep your mask on indoors in public—unless you're playing the clarinet.

WEDNESDAY | AUGUST 11, 2021

I T'S WEDNESDAY NIGHT AND IT'S RAINING (AGAIN), so there go the plans for the first church choir rehearsal of the season.

We're rehearsing out of doors due to the rapid spread of the Delta variant throughout the state. We're pretty much all fully vaccinated, but we don't want to become a case report on an infection cluster, so we figure we'll rehearse outside for now, although that does leave us a bit at the mercy of the weather gods.

Being from Seattle, rain doesn't particularly bother me. I'm perfectly happy to show up in a rain hat and galoshes, but I suppose the pages of our sheet music will start sticking together, especially as we're having these intermittent rain cells where absolute torrents pour down over ten minutes or so before it returns back to its regularly scheduled 90 degrees. As the next hour or so is now unexpectedly off, I might as well write.

There were 3815 new COVID cases reported to the Alabama Department of Public Health yesterday; the seven-day average of cases is 3355. At the peak of the winter surge, our case numbers topped out with a seven-day average of just over 4000 cases, so we're more than 80% there and the numbers show no signs of slowing down. At this rate, by the end of next week, we're likely to have more cases in the state than we did at the peak of the winter surge.

The memos are flying thick and fast at my hospital systems to batten down the hatches again. Transfer visits that don't need to be in person back to telehealth. Reduce scheduled and elective admissions. Prepare to have staff and students be pulled away from their current rotations back to COVID duty. Re-open drive-through testing sites.

Inpatient numbers aren't as dire as they were this past winter—yet. This is likely a function of the elder population having had their vaccines and therefore not falling ill in the numbers that they were this past year. But the numbers are steadily mounting, and I hear every day about another relatively young healthy person who intersects with my circle of acquaintances being hospitalized in an ICU.

The Delta variant which—if we had had better vaccination rates this past spring when vaccine became readily available, wouldn't have become such a concern—continues to rip through the land with spectacular speed. Enough data has come in to suggest that it has an R0 of roughly 7. One infected person infects seven others on average. The original Alpha strain had an R0 of about 3. One infected person infected three people on average.

I've always been intrigued by exponents, so let's look at the difference between the powers of 3 and the powers of 7. Calculators out: 3, 9, 27, 81, 243, 729, 2187, 6561, 19683, 59049. That's enough. Now the other 7, 49, 343, 2401, 16807, 117649, 823543, 5764801, 40353607, 282475249. After ten iterations, the powers of 7 are nearly 5,000 times larger than the powers of 3.

There are only about 5 million people in the state, so it only takes seven or eight iterations at an R0 of 7 to get a number that surpasses the number of people. This is the reason why it's so potentially dangerous and why the numbers have zoomed up seemingly overnight.

The thing I don't quite get is the political doubling down coming from certain quarters of the Republican party. They should be able to do (or hire someone to do) basic math which shows exactly what's happening and why, and that a whole lot of people are going to get sick faster than the health system—already weakened by the first year of the pandemic—can possibly cope.

Rather than quietly abandoning their rhetoric (which they could get away with under the improving conditions of the Alpha strain seen this past spring and early summer) for a real-world assessment of rapidly changing conditions, they seem content to play toddlers standing on the playground screaming "Mine Mine Mine" and "No No No" over and over again.

Part of adulthood is recognizing that the world is the way it is rather than the way you want it to be, and that no amount of magical thinking can change it. Unfortunately, the Republican party has, since at least the time of Ronald Reagan, used a combination of money and naked force to reshape political reality, at least, to their choosing, and they have now made the mistake of thinking that these tactics can achieve success in any endeavor. However, coronavirus is like the honey badger. It don't care.

I was on a Zoom call last night with a group of community leaders brainstorming ways to get vaccine rates up and how to communicate more effectively with various population subgroups. One of the leaders suggested that we all go to various political meetings with a message of vaccine positivity backed by science and our credentials. After seeing news footage of screaming mobs of anti-maskers and anti-vaxxers at school board meetings, city hall meetings, and town halls all over the country, I don't think I want to subject myself to that kind of abuse.

Doctors and nurses and public health workers of all kinds who are just trying to protect their neighbors from irreparable harm are being subject to assault, battery, doxxing, and general bad behavior of all sorts. I have absolutely no idea how you change people who are not living in a world of rationality but in one of emotions and feelings and inflated egos. At least on Facebook, when people don't agree with what I have to say, they have to leave a comment that I have the option of erasing should I so choose. (It's very rare that I have to do that, but I have done it and will likely have to do it again.)

The storms today were reminding me a bit of Tommy.

He and I liked to sit in bed in our old house on the hill and watch the storms race up the Jones Valley. In 2004, when we had been together for about a year and a half, and were just starting to dip our toes together into the Birmingham performing arts community, hurricane Ivan came ashore on the Gulf Coast and headed inland directly over the city. Everything was canceled, the power was out, and we were on the floor of the bedroom playing a prolonged game of Monopoly.

The winds were blowing, the house was rattling, but 200 miles inland, we were unconcerned until we started to hear an odd noise from upstairs in the living room. We went up to investigate and found that the rotation of the winds, being the opposite of the usual prevailing weather, was pushing the rain up under the shingles. Water was pouring into the living room from several points—the only time we ever had serious leak issues.

Of course, one of the major leaks was right over Tommy's precious grand piano, so we immediately had to move it and all the living room furniture into the dining area and fetch every bowl and bucket we could find. The piano survived, although we did have to get a few of the felt hammers replaced. The buckets were enough to prevent further catastrophe.

We finished the Monopoly game, and at seven o'clock that evening set out to see if there was power anywhere nearby. Fortunately, Five Points South was fully lit up so we went out to dinner, had several cocktails, and went to bed early. We decided dinner and cocktails was definitely the best way to end a hurricane and vowed to try and make that a tradition.

Rains-a-comin'-in again, both literal and metaphorical. Hold tight, put up the storm windows, wash your hands, wear your mask, get your vaccine.

SATURDAY | AUGUST 14, 2021

THE NUMBERS KEEP SOARING.

Six weeks into this new surge, we have caseloads and hospital numbers we haven't seen since last January when a new administration and distribution of vaccine finally began to bring numbers down.

The pandemic during 2020 was, primarily, driven by systemic failures in our politics on a national level. The election of an administration that saw itself as a wrecking ball, bent on upending the entrenched ways in which the government does business, led to a situation where federal agencies that keep us safe on a national level were unable to function as designed. The change in administration brought a new culture to Washington DC which, when combined with an efficacious vaccine, completely changed the equation, and we were able to return to a more normal life.

The pandemic during 2021 is not due to a failure of our politics; it's due to a failure of our society.

We have, for whatever reason, decided it is no longer important to care for each other. Selfish behavior has become the order of the day. This has given the Delta variant the perfect opportunity to seed itself in the unvaccinated population and travel far and wide very quickly, bringing us right back to where we were eight months ago.

The federal government hasn't brought this about. The Biden administration has done everything in its power to get the word out on vaccines and to get the resources available to states and localities for both preventive and aggressive care. Some states have been working actively against this—Florida and Texas being the most obvious examples—but they wouldn't be doing so if the majority of their citizens hadn't decided to take a political stand based on "Ignore thy neighbor" and "Love only thyself."

There's nothing new about anti-vaccination and anti-science attitudes in North American culture. Mandatory smallpox vaccination rules caused riots in the late 19th century. There's always been a deep distrust of government and its role in regulating bodily autonomy. There's also nothing new about selfishness as a political virtue.

I suppose one of the reasons all of the great religions focus so much on hospitality and welcoming the stranger and loving thy neighbor is to act as a counterbalance to the selfishness that politics and economics tend to engender. When churches lose that mission and natural pull against those forces, they tend to stultify which is why state churches very rarely succeed. They are two opposing forces and states of mind, a yin and yang of church and state that must figure out a way to coexist for society to be vibrant and move forward.

We're in a moment when a significant number of those rejecting sound science and health principles are allied with certain religious denominations. Many of those denominations, in chasing the prosperity gospel, have rejected the basic tenets of openness to the other, which is very hard for humans to do, in favor of closure and definition of themselves strictly by what they are not rather than what they are.

I don't think this is a particularly good way for them to find continued long-term success. I know how hard it is to accept that those different from oneself have full-fledged, authentic lives. I don't think I really got it until I started doing house calls routinely and was welcomed into homes that were not white middle/upper-middle class. I learned how to see the world in different ways than I was used to. It wasn't easy. I still don't understand the life choices of some of my patients, but I have gotten to the point where I will accept them as being theirs to make and not mine to gainsay or change in any way.

I'm wondering if what we're seeing is the death of the religion of medicine. In the early 20th century, the majority of the population had little to do with organized medicine. Specialty and hospital care were for those few with money or who lived in cities. The majority of the population were doctored and nursed by grandma with some help from a neighborhood GP, if there was one to be found.

Things got a little better between the wars, but the Depression ensured there wasn't a lot of expansion in the health sector. People, for the most part, were born and died at home, many at young ages from what we would consider preventable causes these days. Things changed rapidly, however, in the years immediately following World War II.

The post-war boom allowed for new hospitals to be built and for medical schools to upgrade their training facilities. The new wonder drugs, known as antibiotics, created medical miracles as those who would have previously died at home were successfully treated and cured in these new temples of medical learning, filled with white-coated acolytes.

The idea of American exceptionalism in medicine took root in the culture. People felt blessed and worshiped the stunning achievements that came along from CT scans to organ transplantation to robotic surgery. Doctors were granted incredible social authority, and the idea of "Doctor knows best" inculcated even the most modest of households. Whatever the health system suggested, people tended to obey without question.

Then things began to go wrong.

The health system was sold to corporate America as yet another industry that could be monetized. Doctors became beholden to administrators rather than their patients. New information technologies allowed untrained individuals to access vast arrays of medical information with little guidance about interpreting their findings and the results of their research. A fractured media landscape allowed even the most lunatic of beliefs to find a foothold and an audience in the marketplace of ideas, and to be amplified in the name of "fairness".

There was concern that the temples of healing might cater too much to the wrong sort of people, so funding was diverted from the public health system to more private enterprises where the wealthy might take a cut and ensure a certain exclusivity of entry. It is on to this landscape that COVID, like so many other infectious diseases before it, does its one and only job: move from human host to human host, replicating itself without care for what damage may accrue along the way.

The people ignored the cries of the priests in their white coats as if they were so many Cassandras. They were determined to follow their own personal paths to salvation using the philosophies of everyone for themselves that had become popular in the political and economic spheres.

Then they began to fall sick and came to the temple for healing. But there were too many of them and the temple and the priests, having been neglected, were incapable of meeting their demands. Their language of science, being full of uncertainties, confused the people with their sense of certitude in themselves. And so we are where we are. I don't yet know the end or the moral of the story. It's still being told.

><del>

I'm tired.

I'm going to have to go back on jeopardy inpatient call again as UAB has to recreate the COVID surge teams of last winter. I don't want to have to keep thinking about all this. But it's my reality and here to stay for now.

You know the litany: wash your hands, wear your mask indoors in public, keep your distance when you can. Get your vaccines. The life you save may be your own.

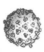

TUESDAY | AUGUST 17, 2021

I SET A NEW RECORD TODAY on my rural house call run: 310 road miles and seven driving hours.

Due to some staff issues, I ended up having to do all the driving myself to Guntersville, Fort Payne, Henegar, and Section. I was a wee bit fried by the time I got back to Birmingham. Notes will need to be written tomorrow as I am in no shape to battle the VA computer system this evening.

I suppose today explains why there aren't more rural house call programs in place. The VA can afford to run a program at a loss as long as it helps the system as a whole. Veterans enrolled in our program have somewhere between 60 and 75 percent fewer hospital days per year than age- or morbidity-matched controls who receive usual office-based care. It doesn't take too many non-existent ED visits or ICU stays to free up enough dollars to pay for house calls.

This doesn't happen a lot in other systems for two reasons. First, in most systems, inpatient and outpatient sectors are siloed from each other financially. There's no way to calculate cost savings between the two realms. Second, there is a dearth of providers out there who feel comfortable with and who truly understand how to provide care in the home environment. One of today's patients was just out of a community hospital in Northeast Alabama and, per the family, that institution went from being relatively quiet last week to a zoo over the weekend due to the impact of COVID patients.

>———

The local news regarding COVID keeps getting worse.

Yesterday, there were two ICU beds available statewide. Today, there are a couple dozen more ICU patients in hospitals than there are staff to man those beds—and the numbers aren't even beginning to slow down.

UAB's inpatient census ticked up another couple dozen overnight. There are more than double the number of hospitalized children than there were at the peak of the surge last winter. Local school districts have only been in session for a few days and already the notices of exposures at school are flying thick and fast.

We're not quite at the level of Florida, where one Tampa Bay school district had over 5,000 students out on quarantine, but I won't be shocked if we get there. Death rates are still relatively low, but that's a lagging indicator. It won't start increasing for another week or two.

There's been a lot of grumbling among physicians and other healthcare workers of my acquaintance about having to take care of the willfully unvaccinated who have deliberately put themselves in harm's way and are not only requiring intense resources, but are also drawing away resources from patients with other conditions. While I get the emotional impulses fueling this (those working in healthcare are exhausted after 18 months of this with no end in sight), I can't agree with it.

My ethical compass dictates that I help patients, no matter the cause of their discomfort or illness.

If we start drawing lines, where do we stop? Do we stop treating lung disease in smokers? Liver disease in alcoholics? Injuries in those at fault in motor vehicle accidents? Heart disease and diabetes in the overweight? You can make all of the "right" choices and you're still

278

eventually going to have something go wrong in your body. I don't think any of us has the moral authority to sit in judgment in that way.

The health system is not empowered to make people get vaccinated. The government really isn't either in a free society. We believe in letting autonomous adults choose for themselves, rightly or wrongly, about all sorts of things. There are some carve-outs for public health purposes, but with the highly polarized politics of the moment, I don't see much of anyone in the governmental arena demanding anything from the entire population.

So what will increase vaccination rates? The thing that has always changed American behavior over the years—capitalism.

Free market forces have already figured out that letting individuals with a potentially deadly infectious disease into your place of business may not be the world's best strategy for economic growth. In addition, if your employees become either chronically or terminally ill, given our peculiar employment-based health insurance system, Wall Street is going to stop wanting to pay for things that are largely preventable.

Private enterprise is going to put more and more rules in place. They will, of course, be challenged in court, but with the packing of the courts in recent years with judges siding with corporate interests over the interests of the individual, I figure the right wing may find itself hoisted on its own petard.

I had a meeting this weekend to start thinking about a possible new version of *The Politically Incorrect Cabaret* for the fall. Some ideas were bandied about, but we were left at the end with the understanding that we had no knowledge of where society would be in a few months in terms of either attending or comprehending satirical entertainment, so we ultimately decided to see how things develop over the next few weeks before making any firm decisions.

If I were writing the show this week, in addition to COVID, I would also be writing about Afghanistan and the situation there. The end game is incredibly sad but was also inevitable as any student of land wars in Central Asia will attest.

The final withdrawal has been a botch. The administration assumed they would have weeks to plan and execute it, not just a few days. My heart goes out to the Westernized urban populations of Kabul and Kandahar and other cities, especially to the young who grew up in a relatively liberal atmosphere and are now going to be pushed into a repressive medieval society they are entirely unfamiliar with.

I can't really think of ways to make either of these topics funny, even with the cutting humor I usually bring to the PIC that makes people laugh somewhat uncomfortably. Ah well, a problem for another day.

Litany in the meantime—in my best Ansager outrageous accent— Vash yer hends! Kip yer mesks ovuh yer nose unt yer mouth! Don't git toooo close. Vaaahkseenate!

FRIDAY | AUGUST 20, 2021

TODAY IS MY EARLY DAY.

I came home after my lunch meeting to do the Zoom meetings I had scheduled. I finished them up around 3 PM and made my list of all the wondrous things I was going to get done with the rest of the afternoon. Next thing I know, it's after 6 PM and I've been asleep on the couch for three hours.

The lizard brain has me going into play-dead mode again, making me save energy for further disasters to come. Add that to the very long and somewhat toxic work week this week, and nothing was going to get done whether I wanted it to or not.

>———<

I'm tired.

No, I think a more correct way to put it is that I'm tired of being tired. The health system is under severe strain again due to the never-ending spread of the Delta variant, and things are rolling downhill. I and what I do are squarely in the way.

We're pivoting back to more telemedicine appointments, online team meetings, virtual house calls, and losing our trainees to COVID surge teams. UAB and the Birmingham VA have got this. Last year taught us all what to do, but everyone in clinical medicine is getting tired and in need of a little R-and-R for rejuvenation.

There's another major difference between what's happening now and what happened last year. Prior to the vaccine and a better understanding of COVID, everyone was at risk of serious complications. Those of us in health care understood that, but for the grace of God, the person in front of us on the gurney could be our spouse, our parent, our child.

Now, the vast majority of those presenting with serious illness belong to a self-selected group who have chosen not to take advantage of some fairly basic preventive measures. It's getting harder and harder to generate empathy as the Delta surge rolls on.

The current local numbers are still running about 3,700 cases a day statewide. In the last two weeks, Birmingham metro has had about 10,000 new diagnoses. The number of children hospitalized has increased 500% in the last month. The state now has the highest rate of child hospitalization in the country.

Statewide, we're technically out of ICU beds, although here in Birmingham metro we're still OK. The US death toll now stands at 628,000, surpassing the Civil War and moving COVID to the second-highest mass casualty event in US history, ranking only below the Flu pandemic of 1918-20.

Exact US casualties from that pandemic are not known. Estimates range from 500,000-850,000 with most coming in around 700,000. We'll be there by the end of the year. In the meantime, the governor and state officials refuse to do much of anything regarding public health measures besides widely ignored suggestions.

The mask wars rage on, especially in the schools where the virus is running rampant. To top it off, the prior president is holding one of his rallies in a cow pasture 50 miles north of town. I doubt there will be a mask in sight, and I won't be a bit surprised if we see an uptick in local cases in a couple of weeks that can be traced to the event. Our wet summer continues. I won't be downcast if it rains tomorrow and all the attendees find themselves up to their ankles in mud. It might be a reasonable metaphor.

Images of the last week—from babies being tossed over the wall of the Kabul airport to get them out of Taliban-controlled Afghanistan, to severely ill people lying on the floor of the main library in Jacksonville waiting to get monoclonal antibody treatments to hopefully keep them out of the hospital, to right-wing extremists frothing at the mouth as they confront school boards, city councils, and public health hearings full of high dudgeon and misinformation—are enough to exhaust anyone.

I gave up television news long ago. I realized it was bad for me. I'm currently giving *Downton Abbey* a rewatch. It's a bit deceptive though. While it's placid on the surface and full of lovely costumes and crisp dialogue, the subtext of a world undergoing wrenching changes from the Edwardian period to the Jazz Age in some ways mirrors our current time.

Part of our problem as a society at the moment is that this process is happening so fast we can't see very clearly where we were or where we're going. All any of us can do is hold tight to the back of the dragon and try not to fall off.

><@

My mother's parents grew up in the society of *Downton Abbey*. They were teens during World War I, emerging into adulthood thereafter as members of the Lost Generation. My grandmother, whose father was a physician in Edinburgh who died young, applied herself to her studies, went to medical school and qualified as a pediatrician going to work in the Lake District caring for the children of the villages there. She was well educated and somewhat fearless. Making her rounds on a motorcycle as a woman in medicine was a bit of a novelty giving her something of an entrée to, but not a place in, "society".

My grandfather, who came from a family of social climbers who had emigrated to South Africa, was sent to England for schooling at 16. He also went into medicine (his father too, was a physician), and was a member of the Bright Young Things set in London. He was a popular extra man at country house weekend parties, being tall, good-looking, athletic, an excellent golfer, and perfectly charming when he wanted to be.

I don't know if he ever spent a weekend at Highclere castle, but he was frequently a guest of Lord and Lady Astor at Cliveden. He eventually met my grandmother when he, too, finished his medical training at the University of Edinburgh.

Various twists of fate brought them to this country in the early 1930s where they settled in San Francisco. My grandmother never practiced after she emigrated. She became the power behind my grandfather's rise at the University of California, all the way to chancellor, and became a friend and beloved mentor to the few women in medical school during the 30s, 40s, and 50s.

My grandfather used his charisma, his erudition, his athletic prowess, and his force of will to succeed. Unfortunately, he saved it all for his professional facade. He was nowhere near as nice a man in private life. But those are stories for another day.

I am supposed to go to Europe in two and a half weeks for my R-and-R.

I keep expecting the trip to be canceled by the tour company or flights to be grounded or some other disaster. It would fit in with this whole crappy year. There's also a piece of me that feels incredibly guilty for wanting to go, that somehow it's a flaunting of privilege in a world of suffering and discontent.

I realize that I am very lucky.

I am not in danger of losing my job. I have enough money to pay my bills. I can even afford a few little extravagances now and then. So many cannot say these things. But I do what I can. I get up in the morning, go to work, and try to save the world entire, one patient at a time. It's all I can handle. And these days, there are times when I'm not sure I can do even this.

Enough!

Time for the Dowager Countess of Grantham and her continuing battles with Mrs. Crawley. They knew a few things then. They washed their hands, kept appropriate distance from others, wore a mask when indicated, and believed in modern medicine.

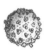

TUESDAY | AUGUST 24, 2021

ANOTHER DAY, ANOTHER SLOP BUCKET full of bad news. The seven-day average of new cases in Alabama is back up over 4,000 cases a day for the first time since the peak of the winter surge in January. US deaths are back up over 1,000 a day. Statewide, we have about 60 more ICU patients than staffing.

The nursing shortage is becoming more and more acute with hospitals frantically looking for and paying top dollar to anyone with a nursing license who is willing to work. I've heard of signing bonuses in excess of $30,000.

Birmingham itself remains relatively resilient as medicine is its major service industry. We have a lot of capacity in terms of both physical plants and staffing but, if the models that have cases doubling again between now and Labor Day hold true, even we will be treating people in parking garages and tents.

The local scuttlebutt passed around physician-to-physician is multiple stories of young healthy people 20-50, who went from the sniffles to full-fledged COVID pneumonitis within a few days and are now fighting for their lives in the various ICUs around town. Nearly all are unvaccinated, either for reasons of politics or inertia. These are the ordinary everyday people who make up the background of our lives: a kindergarten teacher, a school bus driver, a fast-food worker, an apparel store clerk.

A tired workforce of nurses, therapists, physicians, pharmacists, unit clerks, custodians, dietary workers, and all the other people who make up the modern hospital, trudge in for their shifts, hope to win small battles, and look down in anguish when they lose and another once vital young person is no longer here.

One of the things I hear bandied about is the idea of why should we worry, COVID kills less than 1%. Actually, the total death toll to date is closer to 2%, but as the elderly with much higher death rates have gotten vaccinated, the number is starting to fall.

It may be only 1%, but for the people who love each victim, it's a 100% loss. It's easy to write off other people's lives in the abstract, but a much tougher proposition in the concrete when it's someone in whom you have an emotional investment.

I read somewhere once about the shopping cart test.

The way to tell if someone has empathy or consideration outside of themselves is to watch what they do with the shopping cart in the grocery store parking lot once they've loaded their purchases into their car. The empathetic person returns the cart to the cart corral. It's an easy thing to do, requires little effort on the part of the shopper, but does mean that they have to go out of their way a little bit to make someone else's life easier.

The non-empathetic person leaves the cart to fend for itself, uncaring that they've created more work for the person whose job it is to round the carts up and return them to the front of the store for the next go-round.

And there's the issue.

Currently, we've developed a society that not only doesn't return its shopping carts, but also runs over them a few times with their SUV on the way out of the parking lot.

This innate selfishness shows up in many ways. Perhaps the most obvious is the 40-plus-year march to privatize and monetize the public sector which has left our governmental buildings and general infrastructure something of a shambles.

Compare US public/governmental buildings built over the last 40 years to those built in almost any other developed country in terms of architecture, artistry, use of open space, and pleasant environment. I see it most clearly in the VA part of my job. The buildings and offices we work in, as they have had to be constructed on limited budgets, are functional but not necessarily inviting or inspiring of confidence.

Today was an election day locally for mayoral, city council, and school board candidates. All I could think of were the pictures of people waiting in lines hours long to vote in some precincts during the last national election and just what care was taken to design a system to allow that. In my neighborhood, there would be a riot and a rush on city hall by people "who matter" if such a thing were to happen.

I got wind today of a bill making its way through Congress.

The pandemic has ripped the blinders off our national government, exposing something that I have been shouting from the rooftops for the last 30 years. The departure of nurses, nurses aides, and other direct care providers from the healthcare industry is leaving a huge gap in available care for vulnerable and aging adults, just as the Baby Boom is starting into its years of infirmity. Anyone who has looked at a demographic chart for the US created after 1960 has known this would happen; it's just a couple of years ahead of schedule due to the stresses of the pandemic.

The bill in question would mandate a minimum wage of $15 an hour for any person involved in direct care for an elderly or otherwise vulnerable adult. This would include nurses aides, home health aides, sitters, therapy assistants, housekeeping assistants—any of the lower-level positions where someone has to lay on hands in some way.

The theory is that if the wages are improved, more people will flock to these jobs. I don't think it's going to be quite so simple.

The nursing home and home health industries have structured themselves over decades around low wages for these sorts of positions, usually in the $8-10 an hour range. Mandating huge increases is going to put enormous strains on the corporate structures behind these companies. We've allowed this sector to move from not-for-profit to for-profit and, if they can't make a profit, these companies will simply cease to offer these services.

Driving eldercare into bankruptcy just as the Baby Boom is going to require it doesn't strike me as sound social policy. How to balance this? Quite frankly, I don't know.

These are issues that have been predictable and discussed in geriatrics/gerontology quarters for well over half a century. Society, with its focus on youth, hasn't wanted to pay attention. They may be forced into it sooner than I had thought. I was expecting the 2030s to be the decade of eldercare quandaries. It looks like I was off by a few years.

In the meantime, you all know the drill. Wash your hands, stay distant in crowds, wear your mask indoors in public, and get your vaccine.

SATURDAY | AUGUST 28, 2021

AND ANOTHER WORK WEEK COMES TO AN END. One more until I get a much-needed break.

My last time off was in early May, a time of optimism with vaccine being jabbed into willing arms and rapidly falling caseloads. I made the mistake of coming back from that break, driving cross-country to Seattle and back, and setting up what I thought would be a sure bet vacation in which I could recuperate from all of the stresses and strains of the past year. I set it for September, early enough for good weather, but late enough to avoid the crowds. More fool I, having no idea of what was to come over the summer.

I knew that the Delta variant was going to be a risk. I had no idea that half the country would refuse the vaccine and spend the summer eating horse deworming paste. I'm still planning to leave after Labor Day, but I'm clear-eyed enough to know that anything is possible over the next ten days. Who knows if I will get to enjoy a little R-and-R or be stuck with yet another staycation with the cats?

Things aren't looking a lot better since the last time I ran the numbers. Birmingham and UAB are still holding steady at around 175 inpatients with COVID. The number of new cases statewide is now up over 5,000 daily which is the highest it's ever been. Those will translate into hospitalizations in mid-September and deaths at the end of that month.

The lackadaisical attitude toward masking in local school districts has led to up to 20% of the students being out with COVID in some places. Teachers and staff are also getting sick, leading to interrupted instruction, lack of supervision, and a rapid movement of the educators of my generation toward retirement.

The morgue trailers are rolling into the Southern part of the state while the governor refuses to exercise any of her powers and the state Board of Education spends its time trying to protect impressionable young minds from Critical Race Theory, taught only in Ph.D. programs and law schools.

I think the theme of the evening is parasites.

According to my dictionary, a parasite is an organism that lives in or on another organism and gets its sustenance from or at the expense of its host. There's a lot of that going on in society at the moment. One sees it throughout the economic and political system—various and sundry types of people who do little to actually improve the world but who gather their riches from it all the same.

There are those who might say the whole capitalist enterprise is parasitic in nature, with its emphasis on creating wealth from public resources and the labor of others. Certainly, the Marxists among us would have a lot to say about the parasitic nature of the bourgeoisie vis a vis the proletariat. But I am not a trained economist so I'm not going to belabor those points.

I'll start with the most basic of parasites, the biological kind. Ivermectin has been all over the COVID headlines in recent weeks. It's been touted in alternative medicine circles as a cheap and effective treatment for some time, since nearly the beginning of the pandemic.

Ivermectin is an antiparasitic drug that's been around for decades, mainly to treat enteric worms in both animals and humans. I learned about it in med school in association with strongyloidiasis, ascariasis, filariasis, and various other worm-related diseases you've never heard of.

Early on in the pandemic, when research labs around the world were trying various drugs off the shelf to see if anything would work in vitro to inhibit coronavirus replication, ivermectin was noted to work. This finding was rushed to publication and soon picked up by the lay press.

What was not made clear by the initial reporting was that in order to attain the concentrations of drug in a living human that were possible in the test tube, you would have to give doses about a hundred times the fatal dose and that the results had yet to be replicated in vivo. (In vitro means in the lab/cell culture/test tube; in vivo means in a living organism.)

Studies all over the world were done with ivermectin with results all over the map. Some show efficacy. Some don't. There have been significant charges of data manipulation and plagiarism with some studies, causing them to be withdrawn. Let us just say that the jury is very much out, so the FDA is not about to approve it as a treatment.

America's Frontline Doctors (AFD) is an alternative medicine group pretty much frowned upon by most physicians and medical organizations. (One of their leaders, Dr. Stella Immanuel, is going around stating that ovarian cysts are caused by incubi and demon semen.)

AFD picked up on ivermectin and began promoting it, bringing it to the attention of the portion of the population conditioned to react badly to expert consensus and what they view as the elites. The Frontline group then partnered with an online pharmacy to begin writing prescriptions to pretty much anyone who asked. With the help of social media, demand escalated quickly, overwhelming the ability of the group to meet it.

This caused a less sophisticated population with rural roots to realize that Ivermectin was the active ingredient in a number of agricultural products available at your local Tractor Supply. The thing that interests me most about this whole story is the economics. It takes a certain amount of cash to get the word out, set up partnerships with pharmacies, and all the rest of it. Who fronted the dollars and who is making a killing on the back end?

Now on to Afghanistan and the ignominious end of our 20 years of misadventure there. It's hardly the longest war in history. Both the Thirty Years War and the Hundred Years War in Europe far exceeded it, but some of our current boots on the ground there weren't born when it began. Why did we stay so long past all common sense and a decade after the stated objective of removing Osama Bin Laden was achieved?

Again, I believe the answer is parasites. These parasites are contractors within the military-industrial complex who scooped up more than their share of the $2.5 trillion expended over the last few decades. Ending things would have endangered their cash flow, so lots of lobbying was done in DC to protect the status quo which continued until the previous administration set up the withdrawal on the worst possible terms.

I feel very sorry for the young people of urban Afghanistan. All those under 30 who lived in population centers grew up under a relatively permissive society where they could start to realize their potential. The Taliban is going to extinguish this rapidly, but it's not likely to be as easy for them this time around. I expect we will see a good deal of civil war for a very long time.

My last thought on parasites brings us back to COVID and some very dangerous rhetoric that is becoming more and more common from powerful voices. The governors of Texas and Florida, in particular, though they are not alone, have been blaming the spread of COVID in their states on illegal immigration across the Southern border. This is easily debunked.

If immigration were the cause, the highest rates would be in border towns such as El Paso and McAllen but that's not the case. Nor would it explain how COVID leaps hundreds of miles to Florida which has no Southern land border. (I think we'd hear about it if thousands of boatloads of immigrants were descending on the beaches nightly.)

The problem is that the language regarding immigrants is changing and becoming more metaphorical: that they are diseased; that they are vermin; that they are parasites endangering the American citizenry. This language of dehumanization, which equates society with the body and the other as the disease invading it, is one of the necessary steps toward mass murder and genocide.

This has been well studied. If you look up the ten steps of genocide, it's step four. We may like to think it can't happen here, but I don't think the people of Sarajevo at the time of their Olympiad imagined Srebrenica was just over a decade in their future either. My antennae are up, especially if there is any movement towards organized paramilitaries aimed at "defense" against "invasion". That's step five.

Enough negative thoughts for tonight. I'm going to pour myself a glass of wine and find a mental comfort food film, like a cheesy 70s disaster flick or an 80s teen comedy. I'm sure there's something new out there, but nothing I've heard of has really spoken to me for a few weeks. And I'm trying to isolate some outside of work, so I don't get a breakthrough infection just as I'm trying to leave on vacation.

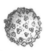

MONDAY | AUGUST 30, 2021

T HIS IS MY LAST WORK WEEK before some extended time off—three weeks with bookending long weekends.

I haven't taken this much time at once since well before the pandemic began. The EU has suggested to its member states that American tourists again become *personae non-gratae* so the planned trip may not come off. I may not even know if things are on until I'm on my way to the airport in a week.

No matter what happens, I'm determined to enjoy myself, recoup some of my energies, and think about what the next activities will be. Get around to some of my home projects that have been languishing? Watch a bunch of movies and write a number of my movie columns on which I am woefully behind? Audition for and book a decent role?

If there's one thing the last 18 months have taught me, it's that I'm terrible at predicting the future, so it's probably not wise to plan too far ahead. Just keep moving, keep breathing, and go with the flow.

The rains of Hurricane Ida are pattering down outside.

No major wind to speak of as we're only getting some of the outer bands here in Birmingham. From what I can tell, all of my New Orleans friends have come through all right, but there's a lot of damage—dormers blown off roofs, trees down, that sort of thing.

I am quite concerned about the state of the hospitals, overcrowded with COVID and no power to speak of anywhere in the New Orleans metro area. The latest estimates I have seen are up to three weeks to get everything back up and functional. The inpatient healthcare workers are exhausted already and additional privations related to power failure may send some of them over the proverbial edge.

The local COVID mask wars appear to be calming down as more and more prominent anti-mask/anti-vaccine personalities fall ill with the Delta variant. The number of news articles I've seen regarding someone of this type being hospitalized with critical illness or having died is heading toward the triple digits, so maybe the message is finally beginning to seep through that defiance of public health precepts in the presence of a highly contagious viral illness may not be the best strategy for a long and happy life. We shall see.

Rumor has it that the hold-out local school district over masking is capitulating. I have certainly seen more and more adherence to masking and social distancing in my journeys around town over the last few weeks. My pharmacist friends also say that they are booking more and more appointments for first vaccine.

I'm trying to think of a good story to tell as it's been a while since I recounted one of the adventures of my misspent youth.

I've told all my personal hurricane stories in previous installments of these diaries so I'll have to think of something else that involves Stormy Weather but without Lena Horne. (I did see her one-woman show on stage in London back in 1984 and she was fabulous).

I am the eldest child. My sister and brother are five and six years younger than I am respectively. In adulthood, that doesn't mean much, but in childhood, it was a bit of a problem as I tended to be in a very different developmental stage than they were. My parents solved some of that by sending me off to summer camp for a few weeks every July to a place that specialized in horseback riding. My mother had been quite a horsewoman as a teen and she wanted her kids to have that experience as well.

The camp I went to was called the Flying Horseshoe Ranch and it was in the Teanaway Valley just outside of Cle Elum. (For those of you who are not Washingtonians, this, of course, means nothing.)

I took to camp life and, although I was physically quite small, I had inherited some of my mother's horsey genes and was quite good on horseback. I came home with a number of blue ribbons from horse shows over the years.

We campers did all of the usual camp things although, as this was the early 1970s, our counselors were a bit more permissive than they might be today.

One year, we had a boys campout/sleep under the stars over-night away from the camp. We were all bussed to a campground on a stream higher up in the Cascades where we were allowed to run around and be little hooligans to work off our excess energy. It was a beautiful day but, that night, there was an unexpected thunder-storm—lightning, pouring rain, and we were all just stretched out under the pines in sleeping bags without a tent in sight.

Most of us crawled under the picnic tables which didn't help a whole lot in terms of keeping the rain off. The counselors (old and wise to 12-year-old me but likely all of 18 or 19) tried to figure out what to do. They decided to get us back to the camp that night. Of course, the bus wasn't slated to return until the next day, so they stuffed us all in the three cars they had available and drove us back.

I still remember being crammed in the back of an early 70s El Camino with nine other 9-12-year-old boys, whizzing down a mountain road in a roaring rainstorm and having a great time—my frontal cortex not yet having developed enough to understand that maybe this wasn't the wisest of ideas. We got back about 2:30 AM, nobody was hurt, and we all had stories to tell each other for the next few days in the ways of twelve-year-olds.

I'm hungry. Going to raid the refrigerator. Remember the litany. Wash your hands. Keep your distance. Wear your mask in public. Get your vaccine. Maybe I can make a campfire song out of it.

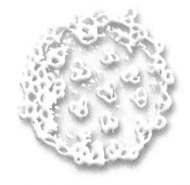

SEPTEMBER 2021

There's No Cure Like Travel

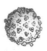

THURSDAY | SEPTEMBER 2, 2021

W E'RE INCHING UP ON 40 MILLION confirmed cases of COVID in the US since the pandemic began 18 months ago. Over the last four weeks, there have been about 4 million new infections and about 27,000 deaths. We're not quite where we were last winter when no one was protected by vaccines but we're rapidly approaching it, and we have certainly surpassed it in the Republican states that have decided basic public health measures are somehow un-American.

Florida, of course, continues to lead the way with numbers blowing last winter out of the water. Texas isn't far behind. Alabama is not doing well, but at least our governor is taking a *laissez-faire* attitude toward tried and true means of spreading infectious disease rather than actively campaigning against them.

The 7-day average for cases in Alabama is now about 15% higher than it was at the peak of the winter surge. How that's going to translate into hospitalizations and mortality in a month or so remains to be seen as it's unclear to me how many of those cases are at risk for serious complications and how many are breakthrough cases in the fully vaccinated.

～☞

The resident I took on my rural house call rotation today just came off the medical intensive care service and had a couple of interesting things to say about it. Last year, residents did not work with COVID cases. Before the vaccine, we were not about to risk the health and lives of young people just beginning their careers. Now that healthcare workers are vaccinated, the risks are much lower and the house staff is working with those patients on those floors.

This young woman mentioned that all she took care of during her month of ICU was COVID. She felt good about handling those individuals but feels that maybe she was cheated out of learning about other medical conditions that require intensive care, everything else having been crowded out.

She also was very interested in the family dynamics of the people she treated. The majority were in their 40s and 50s, previously healthy, and, therefore, had not given thought to their mortality, had prepared no advance directives, and had no discussions with their families about such things as code status, CPR, or final wishes.

Time and again she found herself in the waiting room with their children, mainly high school age to mid-20s, asking them what should be done, and these young people not really being able to comprehend what was being asked of them. They almost always said "Do everything!" because it's their understanding that they should have their parents until they themselves are comfortably middle-aged, and they can't imagine being young without them. They don't really comprehend that "Do everything!" in an ICU situation with a disease that destroys the lungs rarely turns out well for anyone concerned.

I was wondering what I should write about this evening when I ran across yet another news story about ivermectin, the anti-parasitic drug that has caught on as a treatment for COVID. In this particular column, the author was talking about people getting the veterinary version as a topical paste, diluting it with water, then injecting it.

The trained physician in me shivered as there are so many things wrong with this approach that I don't know where to begin. Perhaps people will start rubbing it into their eyeballs next.

As I believe I wrote earlier, there is good scientific evidence that ivermectin blocked replication of the virus in the laboratory. Experiments to show what dose might be appropriate in a living human, and whether it has that same effect in living tissue rather than in cell culture, have begun but have not yet produced any data that would allow the FDA or any other regulatory body to approve the drug for use in the treatment of COVID.

These experiments are in process and, if they show promise, I'll certainly write about it at that time. In the meantime, ingesting topical horse paste or injecting dewormer mixed with tap water is a really bad idea. There are a number of people in ICUs nationwide with liver failure from ivermectin toxicity, taking up those few beds not occupied by COVID patients. Take it from a physician, dying from liver failure is not a pleasant way to go.

⟞⟝

Physicians, with our ceremonial robes of the white coat, descend from the priesthood. We are the intercessors with the gods and with fate who miraculously restore the balance of the world through the healing of the individual. As George R. R. Martin put it, "What do we say to the god of death? Not today."

As these age-old archetypes have come down to modern America, a little of the idea of healing magic has continued to cling around the edges. We're a very literal people. We like our magic to take physical form so we embody it in the prescription.

Most healthy people, when they have need of health care, have developed an acute illness or complaint that has some sort of reliable cure or amelioration. If we're going to take a day off work, drive downtown, spend 20 minutes trying to find a parking space in the overfull deck, wait while the doctor is running an hour or more late thumbing through an old Golf Digest, and then sit in a too cold exam room in our underwear, we figure we better get something for all that inconvenience or we've wasted our time.

The prescription is part of the deal. This is implicitly understood on both sides of healer and patient. We, therefore, tend to imbue the

301

prescription with supernatural powers for good, and we carry that idea of medicine as a good thing with us throughout our lives. When this gets mixed in with our cultural ideal of the quick fix, we lose track of what medications actually are.

Medications are controlled doses of poisons.

What is a poison? A poison is a substance, which when taken into the body, alters that body's balance and physiology to a negative end result. A medication is a carefully measured and tested substance, which when taken into the body, also alters that body's balance and physiology. It's more or less the same thing, only with medicine you trust you aren't going to get that bad thing happening.

Some medications are literally poisons. The most famous example is the drug warfarin (brand name Coumadin) which is used as a blood thinner. It's called warfarin because it was developed at the Wisconsin Army Research Facility (WARF). Its intended use when first invented? Rat poison.

In the 19th century when medications were not regulated, people died from them all the time. The public outcry during the progressive era is what led to the creation of the FDA. It coincided with the Flexner report that helped to standardize medical education.

Society accepted that only trained individuals should handle and dispense medications as they could be dangerous in untrained hands which is why physicians, nurses, pharmacists, and the like, all have to go to school for a very long time and pass innumerable exams to get licensed. Every state in the union has a vested interest in making sure that even controlled doses of poisons are used judiciously with appropriate understanding—something one does not find in social media groups of people hawking outlandish cures.

The biggest issue I have with medications as a geriatrician is convincing older people that sometimes de-prescribing is better than prescribing. Older people, as they sail through life, collect up various ailments and disease processes. It's inevitable. With access to Medicare and an almost unlimited number of specialists, they also collect up any number of medicines to treat these, or the side effects of the original medications (controlled doses of poison, remember).

Sometimes you need to put the ship in drydock and scrape a few of the barnacles off. Geriatricians are comfortable with this. Patients, their families, and most other doctors are not.

There was a great experiment done a few decades ago using family practice residents. The residents sent their older patients to a geriatrician who would then make recommendations for care and send them back to the resident for implementation. Residents are young, impressionable, want to be the best they can be, and take their elders' ideas and ideals as gospel as they prepare to move up in the world. You could see this in this experiment.

If the geriatrician suggested that the resident start a new medication, they did this more than 95% of the time. However, if the expert recommendation was to stop a medication, the resident would only do this about 30% of the time. They would not de-prescribe. De-prescribing is antithetical to how we are trained to think as doctors. It's a concept that's difficult for a brain to wrap itself around, especially if that brain has been trained to hone down through a differential diagnosis to find just what the problem is and just the right medication to fix it.

As the Baby Boom, with its generational love of substances of all types, continues to age, becoming more and more geriatric by the year, it's going to become even harder for me and my colleagues to keep people out of trouble. Not only do we have to worry about medications, we also have to worry about substance abuse, over-the-counter medicines, herbal and other natural remedies, things hawked on late-night infomercials, and stuff patients borrow from their neighbors which may or may not be appropriate for who they are.

The average older person takes seven medications daily (four prescribed, three over-the-counter). There has never been a controlled study published in any language on a human body with more than three drugs circulating in their system at the same time. It's too hard. We have no clue from a scientific point of view what's going on in someone with 7... 9... 16... 25... 41 medications entering the bloodstream daily. That's the art of medicine: and it's more Jackson Pollock than Rembrandt.

It's late. I have an early morning meeting. You know what comes next. Wash your hands. Wear your mask. Keep your distance. Get your vaccine.

MONDAY | SEPTEMBER 6, 2021

IT'S A DOUBLE HOLIDAY TODAY.

Happy Labor Day and thank the union members of earlier generations who fought and died for weekends and the 40-hour workweek.

Union membership as a counterweight to capital built the middle class in this country. It's no accident that the decline of unions following the Reagan administration's union-busting tactics and successful campaign of rebranding unions as parasites in the eyes of voters parallels the decline of the working class into impoverishment.

In addition, La Shana Tova to all of the members of the tribe out there. As a proud Unitarian Universalist, I'm happy to celebrate any religious tradition's holiday that comes along. As we enter the year 5782, I have lots of things to look back on and lots of things to look forward to as well.

Most immediately, I think I've made it through all the hoops and should be able to leave on vacation tomorrow. Fully vaccinated? Check. Negative COVID test yesterday? Check. Passport still up to date? Check. Compression socks to keep the legs from swelling? Check. Forms filed with the Portuguese government so that they can track me down if the wrong person coughs on me on the trip? Check.

I still fully expect something to go wrong and to be turned back at one of the four airports I need to pass through in the next 36 hours. But no one can say I won't have tried.

There's a piece of me feeling very guilty about not having voluntarily canceled this trip, booked in the heady optimism of last May when everything was improving on all fronts. Am I flaunting my privilege? Is it irresponsible of me to be traveling, especially by air, while the Delta variant is running rampant?

I'm not too worried about being exposed during the trip. The tour company is mandating full vaccination for all guests and staff and, given the way things have been going around here, I'm less likely to be exposed in the museums and cathedrals of Iberia than I am in the local Wal-Mart.

Travel journaling plus a look at American society and politics with an outside perspective should commence soon. If I don't make it successfully, I'll take some pictures off my back deck with the cats and we can all pretend they're exotic.

I had dinner with Tommy's parents tonight. We see each other every few months. They're good people and we've worked out an appropriately friendly relationship now that Tommy is gone.

Actually, I've always gotten along better with his parents than he did in our time together. I think deep down he wished that they had been a different kind of people, maybe more like my parents where

I have always been perfectly happy to accept them and meet them where they are.

On the way to and from their house, I had the XM radio on the 80s station. They were rebroadcasting a special they did last month, celebrating the 40th anniversary of MTV which began broadcasting on August 1, 1981 with, as every trivia aficionado knows, the video to the Buggles' *Video Killed the Radio Star.* All of the surviving original VJs were participating along with artists whose videos were played that first day.

I didn't see MTV at its debut. On August 1, 1981, I was floating somewhere in the Bering Sea on a University of Washington research vessel running water sampling equipment. I arrived back in Seattle a week or two later and did some odd jobs before heading to California and my sophomore year at Stanford.

My parents didn't have cable, so the early cable channels were something I enjoyed when visiting the family home of my college roommate, whose father was an executive in the Silicon Valley tech industry and who had all the latest gadgets. I do remember catching MTV with him, his younger brother, and a few others in their family room late that summer and early fall.

The artists that Sirius XM were featuring—Rick Springfield, Huey Lewis and the News, Men at Work, and all the rest—immediately took me back to my undergraduate days, a period of time I enjoyed immensely. I also remember having quite the crush on the young, cute blond VJ Alan Hunter, never dreaming that our paths would actually cross about a quarter-century later. He's a Birmingham boy and we became friendly through both performance and church circles in recent years.

><=

We all lay down the soundtrack of our lives from about the age of 11 to 25. I read somewhere that the pivotal year is the year we are

14. Whatever we are listening to at that time is what we carry in our brain as good music for the rest of our days.

When working with my dementia families, one of the things I encourage them to do is figure out what the patient's musical life was like at that stage and then get recordings of that music and keep them handy. When they're getting restless or agitated, put that on and encourage them to sing along. It usually works, and it's a lot safer than antipsychotic medications.

For my patients who grew up in the country without a lot of re-corded music exposure, it's the old hymns in traditional arrangements that work best. For those who had radios, it's Big Band, Frank Sinatra, Jo Stafford, Patti Page, Dinah Shore, and others of that ilk. When I become demented, which I sometimes feel could happen as early as next week, people better start putting together a mixtape of 70s-80s pop, classic Broadway, the Great American Songbook, and symphonic music of the Romantic era, especially Tschaikovsky.

I'm going to try and get some decent sleep tonight as tomorrow night is a redeye flight and I doubt I'll get much. Got my masks, got my hand sanitizer, got my shots, and I'll try not to get too close to anyone.

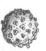

WEDNESDAY | SEPTEMBER 8, 2021

AND SO WE COME TO INTERNATIONAL TRAVEL in the time of the Delta variant.

I wouldn't have booked this trip last spring if I'd had any idea of what was going to happen over the last couple of months, but I did. When push came to shove, I decided on going to Europe, where the population still believes in basic public health measures and community values, and where I was likely safer than in the rural communities of North Alabama where I make my house calls.

What's my general takeaway from a 20-hour travel day involving four airports, three flights, two continents, and one set of lost luggage? Europeans are much better at universal masking than Americans. No one fusses about it, and everyone fills out a whole lot of paperwork so the authorities can find you and get you tested if you're determined to have been in close contact with an infected person. Testing and contact tracing are believed in as general public health tools that have been used for centuries to mitigate epidemic disease rather than as some sort of impingement on "freedom".

I arrived at Birmingham airport yesterday afternoon with plenty of time to spare just to give me some breathing room in case anything went wrong with my sheaf of travel and health documents. The lady at the Delta counter was very nice but thoroughly confused as to what I needed for the various legs of my flight. Apparently, the rules keep changing and they no sooner get training in how to assist passengers when it all proves to be out of date. But I got by: bags checked through to Porto, a quick snack, and then the hop to Atlanta for the trans-Atlantic flight.

We boarded in Atlanta and got settled in our seats. At takeoff time, we didn't. Instead, a phalanx of maintenance guys came down the aisle bearing mops. Not a good sign. The intercom came on in English, and then French with a Chinese accent. My French is pretty good, but I could barely make out every fourth word. The flight attendant responsible for the French announcements was a native Chinese speaker and some of the pronunciations were quite new to me.

One of the aisles was dripping with water. We weren't going anywhere until the source was found, cleaned up, and repaired. The mop guys figured out the problem pretty quickly: a broken water line in one of the lavatories; not something that was going to bring the plane down. They replaced a section of the aisle carpeting and we got underway an hour late.

The long flight was uneventful, save for a closed lavatory on the opposite side of the plane. We arrived safely at Charles De Gaulle airport in Paris, just an hour later than planned. That took my two-hour layover down to one, so it was a quick sprint through a maze of tunnels and concourses to find the domestic terminal. The only real issue was that the airport is designed so that you exit the secure area on leaving the international terminal and therefore have to go through security screening again. Fortunately, the line was moving without too much difficulty.

Then it was on to the next plane for a flight over the Pyrenees from Paris to Porto. Unfortunately, I didn't have a window seat so I didn't get to see much. Porto airport looks like every other midsize city airport you've ever been in. Finally, I headed down to baggage claim to wait for suitcases that never arrived. All of us who had been on that trans-Atlantic flight, about ten total, were without baggage.

The late arrival kept the Delta luggage carts from interfacing with the Air France luggage carts or some such. I have a feeling that any-one on my trans-Atlantic flight who had less than a two-hour layover arrived at their destination sans baggage.

There was a large crowd at the baggage office to register our miss-ing bags (all happily spending a night in Paris). I have been told they will be on tomorrow's flight and delivered to the hotel—unless the flight is late in which case they'll show up on Friday. As I'm here until Sunday, it's all good.

I was met by a lovely young man with a luxurious Mercedes who drove me from the airport into town and to my hotel—the Intercon-tinental—right in the middle of the old city. I got to my room, threw open the curtains, and discovered that my usual luck was holding. I had a lovely view of the construction site next door.

As I had no clothes other than the ones I'd been wearing for 36 hours and had slept in, I located the nearby pedestrian shopping street, wandered up there, and found an H & M and a Benetton which supplied the basics for the next few days. The only thing in the suitcases I'm going to miss is my CPAP machine. It's too bulky for my carry-on. Ah well, I just won't sleep as well tonight as I might otherwise.

I haven't seen a lot of Porto yet. I'll take care of that over the next couple of days. It appears to be a pleasant enough small city, full of Baroque buildings covered with decorative tiles, with red tile roofs being the order of the day. Lots of tourists, so plenty of different languages on the street. I can understand the English, French, some of the German, and some of the Spanish I'm hearing. I haven't figured out the Portuguese yet. I can read it without too much trouble but I haven't figured out the rules of pronunciation.

I'm going to bed early this evening. I will try to sleep as well as I can. That should adjust me for the rest of my sojourn.

Be like the Portuguese: wear your masks, watch your distance, wash your hands, get your shots. Use decorative tiles in your architectural design.

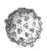

THURSDAY | SEPTEMBER 9, 2021

TODAY WAS A VERY SEATTLE-IN-THE-SUMMER DAY.
Low overcast with temperatures in the high 60s to low 70s.
Perfect for urban walking in the morning and early afternoon.
Drizzle and winds beginning mid-afternoon with the rain getting
stronger and stronger around dinner time.

I have no objection to rain, even on vacation. No native Seattleite
does. If we fussed every time it turned gray and drizzly, we'd never
get anything done in that corner of the world. Just pack your rain gear
and go do it anyway.

The rain showers were likely pushed in this direction by hurricane Larry. My reading of the weather map shows sunshine coming in
the next few days.

I got up relatively early this morning, at least for me on vacation. I
was out on the street by 8 AM. My body hasn't quite figured out what
time zone it's in. That will take another day or two.

The fact that my CPAP was in the lost luggage didn't help. I kept
waking up last night unable to breathe properly. I don't know which
of my ancestors gave me the genes for a soft palate that won't stay
elevated when I'm asleep, but I have a few choice words for him or her
when we meet in the afterlife.

❧

My first stop on my self-guided walking tour was Igreja dos Cler-
gios, an 18th-century church with a 300-foot belfry one can ascend
for views of the entire city. I had hoped that in some 20th-century
renovation they might have installed an elevator, but that was not the
case. I marched up and down all 216 steps. My lungs did not like me
on the way up; my knees did not like me on the way down.

The church was lovely. The view was great. The family of self-ie-taking teenagers from somewhere in the South of France (judging by the accent) was not good company.

Porto is built on the Ria Douro (which means River of Gold if I'm learning my Portuguese correctly). We're close to the Atlantic coast, a mile or so away. I'm assuming the Romans, who founded the city about 2300 years ago, decided that having it upstream a bit on the estuary protected it from Atlantic storms.

The Douro snakes across the Portuguese countryside and into Northern Spain. There are week-long boat tours up and down its length, but not for me this trip. The waterfront is dominated by an enormous wrought-iron bridge, Ponte Dom Luis I, which was designed by Eiffel and various other compatriots in the late 19th century.

The old city is a UNESCO world heritage site. Most of the buildings are 18th and 19th century with baroque detailing and painted tiles. A number are abandoned as the population moved away to the suburbs but, as in Birmingham, a new generation is discovering the positive things about living in reclaimed urban space. There is renovation happening everywhere.

Out of curiosity, I stopped at a real estate office. I could afford a loft here but I don't think retiring to a country where I know no one and don't speak the language is the best of ideas.

Back up the hill from the river and more wandering through commercial and shopping areas. There was quite a lineup outside of one establishment, something one rarely sees at bookstores. Then I realized that this shop, Livaria Lello, was a hangout of J. K. Rowling's when she lived in Porto and was the model for Flourish and Blotts in Diagon Alley. It's dominated by a gorgeous Art Nouveau staircase and a central skylight.

Of course, I had to go in. I bought a copy of the first Harry Potter book in Portuguese and Camus' *The Plague* in the original French. I'll be interested to see if my rusty French is good enough for me to get through it without Larousse by my side.

More window shopping and then, as the rain was strengthening, dinner al fresco in a sidewalk cafe accompanied by several glasses of the local port (named after the city and where the grapes are grown and the wine manufactured). I returned to the hotel to find that my errant luggage had returned from its romantic tryst in Paris, so all is well with the world on this Thursday evening.

✂

Nothing major going on in the world of COVID around here.

The only issue I've run across is that sit-down restaurants are starting to demand vaccine passports on weekends (at least for indoor dining). The unwillingness of the US to do such things means I cannot easily get one. I do have my vaccine card. I can get an insta-test if need be. But it shouldn't be an issue. I am in the hands of Tauck tours as of tomorrow at 1800, and they take care of all that.

Looking at America from a lens of several thousand miles, I noticed that Jim Jordan tweeted that "Real America is done with COVID." That's nice Jim, but COVID isn't done with America.

The numbers keep escalating, the health system is buckling, the schools are a shambles, and all because a once great political party decided to kowtow to science denialism and anti-intellectualism simply to be against what the other side was for.

The Biden administration is tired of letting that minority destroy lives, public health, and the economy for no particular reason. As I write, new mandatory vaccination policies are coming down hard. Cue the howls of outrage in 3... 2... 1...

Bedtime for Bonzo. I haven't figured out what I'm doing tomorrow yet. I'm going to play it by ear. But whatever I do, I have my mask, I have my hand sanitizer, I don't crowd up on people I don't know, and I have had my vaccines.

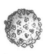

FRIDAY | SEPTEMBER 10, 2021

HAVING ACCESS TO MY CPAP LAST NIGHT after two nights of poor sleep kicked off a chain reaction.

I ended up sleeping for nearly 14 hours. Fortunately, I had nowhere I needed to be or things I needed to do today, so sleeping in and then some wasn't a particular problem. I finally did bestir myself, was somewhat shocked by the time, made myself move, and got outdoors.

The weather was pleasant. Yesterday's rains had gone and we had blue skies. The weather was still relatively cool in the 70s, so it wasn't too hot to amble about.

The first order of business was brunch, a traditional Portuguese combination of espresso, port wine, custard tarts, and something I decided was a combination of deep-fried seafood and potatoes. The server's limited English precluded my being able to discover more. It was perfectly palatable whatever it was.

I headed in a different direction, up the hill to the cathedral, the oldest extant building in town, dating back to the 12th century and Romanesque in style. Gothic arches and flying buttresses had not yet been invented. They came along a century or so later. The cathedral was impressive but not as fancy as others I have been to.

I have always been impressed by European medieval cathedrals. They were generally built over the course of centuries, mainly by individuals who knew that they would never see the completion of their work. They kept at it through war, famine, and plague, for their love of God, culture, and their fellow humans. We could take a lesson or two from them. There's more to life than that which gives us immediate gratification.

Then I climbed across the top of the Ponte de Dom Luis which I had seen from below yesterday. Lovely views, a major plunge to the river far below, and a chance to marvel at the combination of beauty and ingenuity that those of the late 19th century brought to wrought iron. Some exploring of back streets, accompanied by generous helpings of gelato and an occasional glass of port. Then it was time for dinner and a gathering of the tour group.

I had cocktails and dinner with the ten others (five couples roughly five-to-ten years older than I) with whom I will be spending the next two weeks. They all seem pleasant enough. Three of the couples had met on a previous small group tour with the same company in Italy a few years ago and had old home week. It looks like we will all be compatible as we spend the next few weeks together in various hotels, buses, airplanes, museums, and the like.

I am the odd man out, being companionless, but I learned long ago how to be a fifth wheel in polite society, so I don't think it's going to be an issue. Dinner at the hotel restaurant was quite good. I had salmon, well cooked but I suspect farm-raised rather than wild-caught. Being from Seattle, one knows these things.

I have been watching the reaction to Biden's pronouncements on COVID control and vaccination with some interest. I turned on the local Portuguese news to see what they might have to say but found that my understanding of spoken Portuguese was wholly inadequate to the task. I had to resort to various Internet news sites instead.

Reactions from the Republican party and conservative governors, including Governor Meemaw in Alabama, were wholly predictable, and mainly of the third-grade "No one is going to tell me what to do" variety.

I understand this argument, believe me, I do. Bodily autonomy is fairly sacrosanct in terms of cultural mores, the legal system, and medical ethics. Having a governmental entity step up and say "Thou must" is a significant issue.

The question is, of course, where do you draw the lines when your choices in bodily autonomy are causing other people to get sick and die? Does the protection of those individuals and their bodily autonomy and right to life start to outweigh your personal beliefs and choices?

In terms of vaccination, I thought we had settled that a century ago in the Supreme Court's Jacobson decision of 1905. In that 7-2 decision, the court ruled that the state's role in protecting others trumped the individual's right to refuse, and that vaccine mandates were permissible. We've been living with them for years. No one has been too fussy at the wiping out of smallpox, polio, and a host of other feared diseases over the course of the 20th century.

The decision by various forces to politicize the COVID vaccine as a weapon for partisan purposes is something new in American politics. I can't say I'm in favor of it on any level. If there were any proven extreme dangers with regard to the vaccine, I could understand the trepidation, but there really aren't.

Various people state that the VAERS database is full of under-reported complications, but if you look at it, it's a database to which anyone can report anything without any vetting. I suspect that a significant portion of the negative reports are there for political, rather than medical, purposes.

Roughly 200 million doses of vaccine have been administered in the US over the last eight months. The number of serious directly related complications is very small—on the same order of magnitude as being struck by lightning (1/500,000). That's 400 serious complications for 200 million doses.

My publisher continues to be happy with the performance of Volume One of The Accidental Plague Diaries. Apparently, it has been picked up by Target. I don't know if that means it will be available at one near you or if it's just going to be available through their website, but it does mean more exposure.

There's been a bit of a hoorah in the press about Amazon. The majority of their best-selling titles for vaccination (one of my categories) are books full of misinformation and downright lies. This means, of course, that a lot of people are looking at the category. Perhaps they'll see a new book with a sage green cover and some interesting pen and ink art of a medieval plague doctor, and decide to add it to their carts while they are there.

It's all good. I'm not in this to get rich or climb a bestseller list, but I do think there are good and rational perspectives about our trying times that might help others sort out what we have to deal with.

I have to get up tomorrow for a walking tour (likely covering things I have already visited) and a boat tour up the Douro to a port winery complete with tastings. I will wash my hands, wear my mask, and keep my distance while boarding.

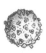

SATURDAY | SEPTEMBER 11, 2021

TODAY WAS LOVELY.

Sunny, no humidity, not too warm. A perfect day for walking tours and boat cruising on the Douro. After my sleep of the dead, the night before, I slept a more normal number of hours and actually managed to make my way down to breakfast.

Portugal definitely works on a different schedule than America. I was finished with breakfast by 7:30, had some time to kill, and went out for a walk. I've always loved walking in European cities. One would think that at 8 AM the streets would be bustling. And yet, they were deserted. Even the local Starbucks didn't open until 9:30 AM.

Some of this might have to do with it being Saturday. Iberian culture breakfasts between 9 and 10, lunches around 2, and doesn't eat supper until after 9 PM. My guess is they don't generally get up much before 8:30 AM for any reason.

><((°>

The first part of the morning was a walk with the group through the old town.

The highlight was a stop at the Church of St. Francis. The exterior isn't much—undistinguished early gothic with a bunch of clashing baroque additions—but the interior is a rococo fantasy of carved wood with every available surface covered with gold leaf carried back from Brazil in the 16th and 17th centuries, half a ton of gold in total.

It's no longer used as a house of worship. It's just a structure to be admired. I liked it very much, but the choice of piped-in music was a tad odd—Schubert's Ave Maria followed by the *William Tell Overture* and *The Waltz of the Flowers*.

Then it was further down the hill to the Douro river bank and onto a boat to see all the bridges from the river's mouth to the highway upstream of town. After that, on to one of the ancient port wineries on the other bank of the river. The one we toured was Taylor's. I've visited many wineries in my day, but this was the first time I'd seen one in continuous operation since the 17th century.

The process of making port wine is somewhat different than table wine. It involves the adding of brandy very quickly in the aging process to stop the oxidation. This is a major reason why port is about 20% alcohol compared to the usual 12% for table wine.

We enjoyed lunch at the winery accompanied by a Fado concert. (Think Edith Piaf songs of longing sung in Portuguese accompanied by guitar.) Then it was back to the hotel, some shopping, and sitting in sidewalk cafes people-watching before turning in. I'll be leaving relatively early tomorrow again as we make our way to Sintra and then to Lisbon.

⌒

I would be remiss if I didn't note that today is the 20th anniversary of 9/11.

I have confused emotions about that day and its images due to its interconnectedness with my own private grief.

Steve had died on August the 1st of 2001. It was not unexpected. He had been quite ill with his interstitial lung disease for some time. I had been taking care of him at home along with his paid caregiver Tameka (who was there when I was at work) and hospice services.

When his battle was over, I decided to take two months off of work with a planned return on the 1st of October. I wrapped up affairs that needed wrapping up, loaded the car, and headed out of town.

I had no itinerary.

I'd been cooped up in the house for a couple of years in my 30s, unable to go much of anywhere other than work. I made a long meandering drive cross-country, using the opportunity to connect and reconnect with friends, eventually ending up in Southern California where I scattered Steve's ashes in the Anza-Borrego desert, his favorite place on the planet. I then headed north to Seattle to spend some time with family, arriving in early September.

On September 11, 2001, I was at my brother's house, sleeping in.

He was at work. My sister-in-law was downstairs with my then two-year-old niece dealing with toddler breakfast things. She flipped on the news, shrieked, and then yelled up the stairs that I had to get up and see what was happening. She and I stayed glued to the television all morning, watching the drama unfold as the towers burned and collapsed.

319

Over the course of the next week or so, I flew to Alaska to see my old college roommate. I had been slated to fly out on the 12th but that didn't happen. I was delayed for several days but eventually did make it to Anchorage and back. Then I drove back across the country, ending up in Manhattan about two weeks later.

The haze was still in the air. The flyers were still affixed to walls. The smell, a mixture of burning electrical systems and pulverized stone, was endemic.

I mourned for Steve. I mourned for the ugly scar in my beloved Manhattan. I mourned for the thousands dead and tens of thousands whose lives were uprooted by the tragedy.

Even to this day, I cannot separate my grieving for Steve from my grieving for the country.

I had hopes that such a national tragedy might unite us and make us stronger. Instead, as we all know, those sentiments were hijacked by the military-industrial complex into fruitless conflicts across the globe which made elites wealthy and drained national wealth away from poorer classes, exacerbating the economic conditions which leave us so riven.

I was wondering today what Steve might have made of my trip to Portugal. He would have complained about the food. (Fortunately, McDonald's is close by; I could have sent him there). He would have complained about too much walking on cobblestones. He would have loved the weather and the boat ride.

He could have done without the winery. He was 17 years sober when I met him, 30 years sober when he died, and prouder of that accomplishment more than anything else.

Tommy, on the other hand, would have loved the winery. He never passed up a winery or a wine tasting if he could help it. As a super-taster, he could identify all of the notes in a good wine. I can't do it and he would always make fun of me for that genetic imperfection.

The only time I remember him having an issue with wine was on one of our trips to Northern California. We drove up to Napa. He was in a snit about something (at this point I have no idea what). Even though we stopped at several wineries, I could barely get him out of the car, and he was sullen in the tasting rooms. Even a little alcohol in his system didn't help. He made up for it on other trips where we went out of our way for Washington and Oregon wineries. Biltmore Vineyards in Asheville, NC was a habitual stop.

Enough for tonight. On to the morrow. I have my hand sanitizer, my masks, and my CDC card all ready to go in my day bag.

SUNDAY | SEPTEMBER 12, 2021

TODAY WAS A LONG DAY OF BUS RIDING.
Down the length of Portugal from Porto to Lisbon with a number of stops along the way. You would think this would be an interminable journey, but Portugal is about 2/3 the size of Alabama, so it was a slightly shorter drive than Birmingham to Mobile.

It was another night of somewhat indifferent sleep for me. Apparently, Saturday nights in Porto are spent having drunken singalongs in the wee hours of the morning under other people's hotel windows. I eventually figured out that housekeeping had not closed my windows properly behind the blackout curtains. When I was able to get that issue rectified, it quieted down somewhat. Although I could still hear the serenades and various other noises until about 4 AM.

After breakfast, the eleven intrepid guests on the tour, our guide, and the driver, headed across the Ponte Maria toward points south.

Our first stop, an hour or so out of town, was the small town of Avenida. Close to the Atlantic coast, it has a series of canals that were used in times past to ferry sea products to storage and processing. Now it's a tourist attraction.

We stopped, took pictures, used the facilities as necessary, and then a little further down the coast to Costa Nova, a Portuguese fishing village that has become a summer resort with all the fisherman's cottages painted in bright stripes and turned into Air BnBs.

Then, one more drive of about an hour to another resort town, Pastais, which has a lovely beach, the usual shops, and restaurants one finds in any beach town anywhere in the world. Stop for lunch—delicious Portuguese-style salted sea bass caught fresh and some sort of spice-pear upside-down cake which was also very good. Then another hour or so, with pretty much everyone sleeping off their postprandial torpor, except our bus driver. Then on to the town of Sintra, just west of Lisbon.

Sintra is built on the sides of an extinct volcano. I imagine it belongs to the same chain as the Azores, Madeira, Vesuvius, Etna, and Santorini. Due to its height and its position near the ocean, it receives the Atlantic winds and is considerably cooler than the surrounding area. Here the Royal family and nobility of Portugal built their summer palaces, places to escape the heat, crowds, and plagues of Lisbon.

We toured the Royal Palace, a hodgepodge of buildings built over six centuries such that no wing lined up with any other. Beautiful tile work, painted ceilings, and an enormous kitchen dominated by two huge conical chimneys towering over the rest of the complex.

As we drove into town and I saw the royal summer palace building, I immediately recognized it. My maternal grandmother had an etching of it hanging in her dining room when I was a child. I had completely forgotten this until I saw those unmistakable chimneys appear.

I have no idea if Lisbon and Sintra meant something to my grandparents. They were European and certainly could have taken a holiday there sometime in the 1920s from the UK. It's a story that never made its way down to me. As much as we would like, not every reminiscence makes it to every generation which makes the ones that do survive all the more precious.

Then it was on to Lisbon, where we are staying at the Ritz, perhaps the poshest hotel room I've ever had the pleasure to inhabit.

There appears to be some sort of diplomatic group from a French-speaking African nation on my floor. Many distinguished gentlemen in expensive suits coming and going. A bodyguard is parked on a chair in the hall just down from my room.

While the interior of the Ritz is sumptuous, the exterior looks a bit like a 1950s girls' dormitory from an undistinguished state college. I'm assuming the building was repurposed in some way from a more pedestrian use. The only issue this time around is that the electronic lock on the door refuses to recognize my key.

They've switched it out three times and it still isn't working. The front desk is getting tired of escorting me up with the master. I heard someone futzing with it a while ago. We'll see if it works in the morning or if I end up locking myself out again.

The Ritz overlooks a large city park. Parque Eduardo VII was named after Edward VII of England who helped strengthen the ancient English/Portuguese alliance (dating back to John of Gaunt's daughter marrying into the Portuguese Royal Family) in the early 20th century. Currently, it's the site of the famous Lisbon Book Fair.

If I had done my research properly and realized this was going on at the time I was here, I might have had some copies of *The Accidental Plague Diaries* sent over and handed them out. I couldn't do that, but I did have a copy with me and could not resist running down and having some pictures taken with the signage.

It's the weekend.

News from Covidland has been quiet and it's late, so I'm going to wind this up now. Spending a long day tomorrow exploring Lisbon, then on to Spain on Tuesday.

MONDAY | SEPTEMBER 13, 2021

IGH-THREAD-COUNT EGYPTIAN COTTON SHEETS, a great mattress, and a quiet room on the 10th floor of the Lisbon Ritz, far above street noise, meant a good night's sleep and up for breakfast with more adventures to come.

The intrepid eleven were on the bus at 8 AM and headed into the old part of downtown for a brief orientation to the city, and then a drive out to the port district of Belem for a stop at the national maritime museum (much devotion to the 15th- and early 16th-century Portuguese voyages of exploration launched by Prince Henry the Navigator) complete with a collection of the Royal river barges. Then along to the Palace of Ajuda, the Lisbon home of the Braganza dynasty of Portugal during most of the 19th and early 20th centuries until they were shown the door in 1910.

The Palace of Ajuda is contemporaneous with Buckingham Palace and has the same general neoclassical proportions. The staterooms are lovely, the banquet hall impressive, and the wandering around between various suites through the servants' corridors gave a feeling of *Downton Abbey* mixed with *The Crown*.

The Portuguese abolished their monarchy a few years prior to World War I, a little earlier than most of the rest of Europe. They had a republic for a while and then a dictatorship under Salazar parallel-ing that of Franco in Spain. In the 1970s, Spain restored their consti-tutional monarchy. Portugal did not.

I looked up the heir apparent should that happen. He's a descen-dant of some second cousin of the last king, there being no direct line left. I don't see him being plucked from obscurity and installed as a monarch at any time in the near future.

After the Ajuda tour, we were turned loose to spend the rest of the day as we wished. I wandered through downtown Lisbon for a while. Not all that different from the downtown areas of other major world cities. I then headed into the old quarter to see the cathedral and to climb the hill to the castle of St. George on the summit, begun by the Moors, and chief defense of Lisbon against invasion by both land and sea for several centuries.

The cathedral was unimpressive—a rather blocky Romanesque affair without much in the way of decoration. The original cathedral was destroyed in the great Lisbon earthquake of 1755. The one that stands was painstakingly rebuilt shortly thereafter to the original plan using what could be salvaged of the original materials.

The castle was more interesting with its original fortifications full of arrow slits, murder holes, and the like. The view from the castle over the town and the Tagus river was such that it was immediately obvious why it was such a strategic location.

Walking up the hill, I stumbled across some partially excavated Roman ruins, part of an amphitheater, and a building whose walls were originally constructed as a public bath. I imagine that if they dig under the castle—below Christian, Moorish, Roman, and Phoenician layers—they'll probably find some ancient Celtic or Iberian settle-ment. It's interesting to think of places being continually inhabited and built upon for thousands of years when in most locations in the

US, it's rare to find anything more than 200 years old.

Finally, a long walk back to the hotel for a nap and dinner.

The news in Portugal today was that they have successfully vaccinated more than 75% of their population and should be up to 85% in the next month.

Cases are falling and the government is relaxing outdoor masking mandates but keeping indoor ones. This is allowing more and more types of businesses to open up. Nightclubs are next, expected in another two weeks.

We could be there in the US but we're not.

Alabama's vaccine rate remains stuck at around 40%. I feel safer here with masks and common sense than I do at home.

I've been watching the continued debate over vaccination in the American press. It looks like the general consensus is that government-mandated vaccination is not overly popular due to the various bodily autonomy/civil liberties arguments.

The Biden administration appears to have threaded the needle. They're not mandating vaccination of all adults, they're mandating vaccination of those employed by the federal government and those who receive funding from the federal government through contracts and programs. That's likely within their purview, especially given years of Supreme Court precedent.

They are also mandating that workplaces be safe under OSHA. Companies with more than 100 employees have the option of either vaccinating employees or testing them weekly to protect other employees with whom they may come into contact.

The other consensus that seems to be gelling is that mandating vaccines to access life's necessities (like the grocery store) is not necessary, but that it's perfectly OK to mandate vaccines for life's little luxuries (air travel, sporting events, theaters, etc.)

I think we're going to be in for a year or two of carefully choreographed compromises like this where those who willfully do not choose vaccination will be tolerated but will find their lives more and more circumscribed. Is this a proper strategy? Only time will tell. It is likely to be accelerated by commercial health insurers demanding vaccination for access to their products.

The thing that gets left out of this strategy is what to do about that small portion of the population that cannot be vaccinated for significant medical or other reasons. If we all stepped up, got our shots, and had a 75% or 85% vaccination rate, herd immunity would start to kick in, and they would be protected without vaccination. With a 60% unvaccinated rate, this just isn't possible.

Tonight I'll celebrate the Portuguese achieving their 75% milestone. But I've still got my mask, my washed hands, my distance kept, and my vaccines injected.

TUESDAY | SEPTEMBER 14, 2021

TODAY'S LEITMOTIF HAS BEEN CLASSIC MUSICAL/FILM. We all had to get up at an ungodly hour in order to catch the early plane from Lisbon to Seville. I'm not sure why we didn't take the bus as they are only just over 200 miles apart. By the time we got through the flight process, arrived at our hotel in Seville, and had lunch, the bus had arrived with our luggage on board, and it was stowed away in our new rooms.

The new hotel is another 5-star Fancy Schmantzy place called the King Alfonzo XIII. It was built to house the well-heeled and the dignitaries who came to Seville for their World's Fair in 1929. It's all marble and tile and Moorish influences, although my favorite parts are the original elevators, mirrored on all four sides, giving a bit of a Willy Wonka vibe to trips up and down from the lobby.

The room is comfortable. I have a view (but no Cockney Signora manning the desk). The bathroom has adequate water pressure in the shower. I am a happy man.

As I was standing in line in the Lisbon airport, waiting to board our prop plane puddle-jumper, it was dark and foggy with a misty rain. I had my envelope of letters of transit from Lisbon. Boarding pass? Check. COVID clearance? Check. Entry card for Spain? Check. All I could think was how Victor Lazlo can you get? Or maybe I'm Ilsa. I suppose it depends on the day.

The short flight went without incident. The rain in Spain was mainly on the plane, and we were motor-coached from the soggy Seville airport into the heart of the city. As we were sitting around the hotel bar waiting for our lunch, it occurred to me that I am making this trip with five married couples, a sort of Iberian bus and truck of *Company*. I wanted to suggest an impromptu of *Side by Side by Side* in the lobby, but I don't think it would have gone over terribly well.

After lunch, I enjoyed a horse-drawn carriage ride through the historic center of Seville, a town of Moorish-influenced architecture, winding streets, pleasant public gardens with flocks of wild parrots chattering away in the trees, and a placid river. After the carriage ride, I spent a lovely few hours wandering through historic neighborhoods, poking into shops, and stopping for the occasional gelato.

At the end of the day, as I was having my third gelato in the cathedral square and the sun was setting, I did some people watching and had a true *Here We Are Again* Leona Samish moment. (Kudos to any of you who pick up on that obscure reference). We have a formal tour of the cathedral and some of the other historic buildings tomorrow, so more on them later.

It's been interesting comparing the general societal response to COVID measures here as they differ from home.

Indoor masking is universal. Outdoor masking is common in crowded situations but isn't done when just walking on the street unless you want to. People pop on their masks without fuss when approaching others or entering a building. There's a general sense of this is what we do for each other as we're all in this together.

High rates of vaccination here are leading to the relaxing of rules, but there's no sense of a wish to race out and push boundaries, rather just one of cautious optimism tempered with an understanding that things need to be studied and rules adjusted constantly around science and data.

Meanwhile, at home, when the science is uncertain and recommendations revised as new data comes to light, people take those uncertainties as a failure of science rather than the result of the scientific method. Instead of absorbing and coping with change, we decide that our own preconceived notions or gut feeling must therefore be more correct.

The latest thing to take off in domestic circles is oral ingestion of Betadine (iodine-based antibacterial goop) as a prophylactic. Kids, do not try this at home. It's highly toxic and we've got enough people in the hospital without adding more poisoning victims.

I will have to change my shoes tomorrow.

My usual walking shoes have worn soles, and much of the pavement in Seville is of marble or polished cement. This, combined with rainwater, has made balance somewhat precarious. I really don't wish to be rushed to Seville General with a head injury. My sneakers have decent tread, so I'll use those instead.

I can see a need to take some of my own advice and pack a

walking stick for cobblestones and other uneven ground in another decade. I'm thinking of a gnarled wizard's staff and a pointy sun hat to go with it.

But now, I'm going to turn in. David Lynch's *Dune,* dubbed into German for some reason, is on TV. This should be a proper distraction as I get sleepy.

WEDNESDAY | SEPTEMBER 15, 2021

T HE WEATHER HELD TODAY.

The storms kept the temperature down in the 70s which was quite comfortable for touring. (My pedometer is most happy with me this week). The humidity, however, has been a bit above my comfort level, though not nearly as bad as Alabama in August.

This morning started with the usual upscale hotel breakfast buffet. Lots of choices and always something that appeals, but European scrambled eggs tend to be runny, and every country does bacon and sausage somewhat differently.

The highlights of this morning's tour were the buildings constructed for the 1929 World's Fair, most of which remain standing around a large public park. We glimpsed them on yesterday's carriage ride, but today was a chance to get a bit closer to see the detail, especially on the monumental Spanish pavilion and plaza.

I had my picture taken with the medallion honoring Don Quixote and couldn't resist serenading my tour mates with a few bars of "I am I Don Quixote, the Lord of La Mancha." I've always been partial to the Don and his tilting at windmills as I have spent a good portion of my life doing the same thing metaphorically.

Then it was back to the center of town for a tour of the largest Gothic-style cathedral in Europe. The nave and chapels are impressive in terms of sheer size and there is some decent artwork including large Murillo and Goya paintings. After the cathedral, we took a ramble through the winding streets of the old Jewish quarter, empty of Jews since the pogroms of 1391.

Per our guide, there are still almost no Jews in the city, fewer than 100 total at the last census. Recently, the Spanish government has had a case of the guilts over the expulsion of the Jews in the 14th and 15th centuries and, if you can prove Sephardic Jewish ancestry back to Spain at that time, you can claim a visa and a path to citizenship.

Given the craziness of our current politics, if I could do such, I might consider it, but I'm about 100% Anglo-Saxon/Celt. I am eligible for a Portuguese "Golden Visa" where, if you purchase real property in the country and bring a certain amount of wealth in, they'll allow you to emigrate. I'll keep that in mind just in case our politicians continue to drive us over the cliff.

My mother was the child of two British citizens living abroad when she was born and could have claimed British citizenship if she chose. With a good lawyer and a great deal of money, I might be able to do so as well, but with Brexit, I'm not sure that would be much of an improvement over my current living situation.

⤚⊙

We then boarded the bus and headed out into the country to a 16th-century hacienda, lovingly restored as an event venue. The location, between the motorway and an aerospace factory, was not promising, but the strategic placement of walls and the opening out of other areas to country views made it pleasant.

There was an entertainment program featuring a flamenco dancing horse (I did not know they had such things) and a leisurely tapas lunch followed. Then it was back to town where I used the rest of my afternoon to visit the Alcazar, the Royal Palace of Seville—still in use as a royal residence if the King comes to town. Very Moorish in its architecture and design but it would be a trifle uncomfortable to live in as it's nothing but stuccoed brick and tile. It has its own private gardens walled off from the city parks that abut it, full of fountains, flowering trees, and bushes. The plants remind me a lot of Southern California—oleander, lantana, jacaranda, bougainvillea, banyan trees, and the like.

We passed a grim milestone today.

The 665,500 US deaths over the last 19 months mean that 1/500 US residents have died from COVID. That's 0.2% of the population. And it does not include those who recovered but who still have significant health conditions. It's roughly the population of Boston.

This means that none of us has a life that has been untouched by the disease. All of us have now lost a family member, friend, or acquaintance. And still, a significant portion of the US population remains mired in a bizarre sort of denial: denial of the disease, denial of the risks, denial of expert opinions.

Here in Europe, denialism exists but is a fringe minority opinion. The majority accepts common-sense advice like masking, hand washing, social distancing, and vaccinations as something we all do for each other so we can live as normal a life as possible. Rates of infection are therefore somewhat lower and, quite frankly, I feel like I am far less likely to run into issues here than at home.

If I didn't have patients depending on me, I'd be tempted to stay a while longer. I could get used to a life of 5-star hotels, cathedrals, chateaux, and a populace that actually culturally cares about each other.

It's back on the bus in the morning, heading for the UK, or at least a little outpost of the UK known as Gibraltar. I'm betting the Gibraltarians wash their hands, wear their masks, and keep their distance.

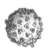

THURSDAY | SEPTEMBER 16, 2021

W E ALL SAID GOODBYE to the King Alfonso XIII hotel in Seville early this morning, boarded the bus, and were soon headed out of town in a southeasterly direction.

Seville may be a port city but it's a river port, about 50 miles inland on the Guadalquivir river, and we were bound for the coast. Our route led across arid agricultural plains, through olive groves, the ever-present citrus, and occasional fields of corn and cotton.

Closer to the coast, the terrain became hillier, with limestone outcroppings. We passed through a large nature reserve, supposedly home to deer and antelope, but they were not posing for tour buses by the side of the road. We topped a final rise, and there, spread out, was the Mediterranean, blue and calm with a large lump on the horizon which we were assured was the Rock of Gibraltar.

Half an hour later, we were in the customs/border control line, getting new stamps in our passports thanks to Brexit, and boarding a minivan for a tour of the rock and surrounding town.

Having a very British mother, I've heard of Gibraltar all my life and have always wanted to see it. Of course, my mother's knowledge of Gibraltar ended somewhere around the Battle of Trafalgar and the death of Lord Nelson during the Napoleonic Wars, so I really didn't know what to expect.

The rock itself, a huge limestone outcropping on the edge of the seacoast, has roughly the same footprint as Central Park in NYC, although it rises to about 1400 feet as a very steep cliff on the east and a bit more gradually on the west.

The old town of Gibraltar and its fortifications cling to the base, rising to about a quarter of the way up the west side, with multiple bastions from the 15th through the early 20th centuries, and topped by a Moorish castle dating back to the 11th.

Various sea powers dating back to the Phoenicians have recognized that Gibraltar is the key to controlling the straits of Gibraltar and passage between the Mediterranean and the Atlantic. This is why the British, awarded the fortified town by the treaty of Utrecht in 1715, have never wanted to give it up, much to the disgruntlement of the Spanish.

Franco closed the border for most of the 60s and 70s which didn't exactly please the Gibraltarians, so they held a plebiscite in which more than 98% of the residents voted to remain British rather than to join Spain.

Over the last few decades, enterprising Gibraltarians, a mix of various European people whose language and culture are British, have filled in some of the bay around the base of the rock, offering more land to build on. There are now gleaming new high rises and other supportive structures allowing the population and economy to expand.

There is still a lack of space.

The one land road into the territory crosses the tarmac of the airport and has to be closed every time a plane takes off or lands. There is a new road being constructed with a tunnel under the runway to hopefully solve that problem in the near future.

Apparently, the airport is one of the most dangerous in the world, not because of errant traffic on the runway, but because of the crosswinds coming in off the Atlantic, spun in unusual patterns by the bulk of the rock. Frequently, flights have to be diverted to Malaga in Spain, about an hour or so away.

We met David, our guide, and a native Gibraltarian, in our small bus suitable for the narrow roads on the rock. It was interesting hearing him switch back and forth from Spanish to English with an East End accent, but that appears to be what the natives do.

We drove through the town and began the zig-zag ascent of the rock over a series of progressively narrower and steeper roads. We stopped at Europa Point, the southernmost point in Europe, and admired the coast of Africa across the strait (roughly 8 miles away), my first sight of that continent.

Then, climbing higher, we stopped at St. Michael's, one of the many caves within the limestone of the rock. Waiting for us there was one of the famous troops of Barbary Macaques, tailless monkeys brought over from Africa as pets that have flourished in the wild. They were bored by our presence (other than the one that reached down and stuck one of his paws into one of my tour mate's ears), so we entered a lovely cave full of stalactites and stalagmites.

I could have done without the tacky *son et lumiere* show in one portion, but the rest of it was quite spectacular. Then, more monkeyshines and a drive back down to the village for a lunch of fish and chips.

After lunch, we made another drive up the coast to the resort town of Marbella, where we are to spend tonight and all of tomorrow as an R-and-R day of sun and surf at our halfway point.

Marbella is a lovely little town, obviously on the upscale end of the Costa del Sol, with a paved esplanade along the water, whitewashed buildings in the original old quarter, and any number of fine hotels, white tablecloth restaurants, and boutiques selling jewelry, resort wear, and assorted bagatelles one finds in beach towns the world over.

I stuck my toes in the Mediterranean (the first time since my trip to Italy and Barcelona in 2002), took a dip in the pool, and had a light dinner with a very large gin and tonic while watching the sunset.

At the moment, I am typing this on my ocean view terrace at the Dom Pepe Real Melia, listening to the vocalist from the restaurant below me massacre her way through the pop hits of the 70s and 80s.

I am looking forward to sleeping in tomorrow and having no agenda—other than keeping my hands washed and wearing my mask indoors.

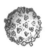

FRIDAY | SEPTEMBER 17, 2021

TODAY WAS A DOWN DAY.

We're just a little over halfway through the tour. It's been fairly busy, so a day without an agenda or having to get on a bus was welcome indeed.

I can't help but think that Fernando, our guide and general herder of cats, and Armenio, our bus driver, quite skilled at maneuvering a full-size Mercedes tour bus through narrow European streets, needed a day away from the intrepid eleven.

Today was about swimming pools, beaches, walks on the esplanade, and a couple of naps. A number of us also got together at a beachside restaurant for a lunch of paella and other treats, and the whole gang had dinner tonight in the hotel restaurant, mainly steak, although I opted for pork loin as I'm not much of a beef person.

Today was the first day on this little jaunt that I felt a bit lonely.

My travel companions are kind and gracious. They make sure I am not left out in any way, but there are times when, as in *Side By Side By Side,* it's obvious there's an empty place next to mine.

Tommy's been gone long enough now that I think I'm more or less over my acute grief and, while I am not looking for a new romantic/intimate partner, I am starting to feel the need for some reliable activity/travel/shenanigans companions with whom I could share an occasional adventure.

I'm sure someone will turn up at the right time. One thing I've learned from life is that things usually fall into place when you don't look too hard and don't force them.

><>

I went through a backlog of UAB emails earlier today and caught up on the local COVID statistics.

The number of folk hospitalized at UAB has been trending down over the last ten days or so which is a good sign. The percentage requiring ICU care, however, is not declining at the same rate. I'm hoping this means that Birmingham, at least, with its significant healthcare worker population, will be on the downside by the time I get back to work.

The various trackers I follow show that this cooling down is likely occurring in urban Alabama. Rural parts of the state, where vaccine hesitancy is so much higher, continue to be hot spots. Vaccine numbers continue to trickle upwards, but the damage done to public understanding of vaccines by politics remains extensive and difficult to overcome.

The FDA met today and came to what I think is a reasonable decision on booster shots: not necessary for most healthy younger adults but appropriate for adults over 65 and for those with significant immune system issues.

How this will be rolled out to the general public remains to be seen but I imagine older adults will be able to receive a booster from most pharmacies, no questions asked and no payment necessary as of the first of the month, maybe even as early as next week. As far as significant immune system issues go, if you don't know what they are, you probably don't have one, so don't worry about it.

><>

Then there's the gathering in DC in protest of the prosecution of the January 6th protesters. Who knows where that will end up?

As I read the European perspective on American political news, I'm tempted to take my retirement savings and purchase a golden visa for resettlement in the EU where people still look out for their fellow countrymen, instead of being at each other's throats.

Of course, the Catalonians and the Castilians might disagree with me on that one.

The bar singer below my window is busy destroying Elton John. I have *The Last Action Hero* dubbed into Spanish on the TV. And there's a lovely moon out, so I'm going to sign off now and drift off to sleep.

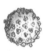

SATURDAY | SEPTEMBER 18, 2021

HAD BREAKFAST AS THE SUN ROSE over the Mediterranean, promising another lovely day on the Costa del Sol. However, I and my traveling companions had a schedule to keep, so it was back on the bus.

We left the environs of Marbella and soon found ourselves climbing a winding mountain road over the original Sierra Nevada Mountain Range which backs up along the Spanish coastline. At first, we were winding through neighborhoods of opulent villas, reminiscent of Malibu or Bel-Air. The occasional Lamborghini or Maserati cruising by completed the picture. Eventually, we were far enough away from the sea that the cars turned into Renaults and Peugeots.

We passed over the crest at about 3000 feet in one of Spain's National Parks which amounted to forests and the occasional white-washed village. We then descended into an agricultural plain, mainly ranching rather than crops, and were soon in Ronda, a fortified town on top of a bluff riven by a canyon formed by the Guadalevin river.

Inhabited since it was first settled by the Celts, centuries before the Romans, Ronda has been fortified, fought over, changed hands, and been the scene of general mayhem many times over the years, most recently during the Spanish Civil War when the Fascists and the Nationalists spent their time tossing each other into the gorge, an episode made famous by Hemingway in *The Sun Also Rises*. Now it's relatively peaceful and sleepy, besieged only by hordes of tourists who come to see the gorge, explore the old town, and thrill to the famous bull ring, continuously operating since the early 18th century.

We peered into the gorge, took in the stunning views of the Sierra Nevadas, had a guided tour of the back ways of the town, and ended up in the bull ring, Pepe our local guide being something of a bull-fight fanatic. One of my trusty New Balance sneakers decided to separate from the sole halfway through the walk and detached completely in the middle of the bull ring. I'm sure there's an omen in that, but I don't think I want to know what it is.

After a leisurely lunch (I had oxtail stew, the local specialty) at the edge of the gorge, we were back on the bus for a few more hours until we reached the old Moorish city of Granada. I was on the fatigued side, so I did not explore much beyond the immediate surroundings of our hotel as we will be here tomorrow as well.

Our hotel, the Alhambra Palace, is on the same hill as the landmark itself (being visited tomorrow morning) and has the same spectacular view out over the city. The hotel was apparently designed and decorated by the same people who created the great Moorish 1920s movie palaces in the USA and is delightful in a rather Arab kitsch fashion. Can't beat the views though and the room is comfortable, although I'm not sure what to make of the combination toilet-bidet that has a control panel more suitable to the Space Shuttle than a bathroom fixture.

I'm afraid to push too many buttons.

We all met up for dinner at a charming restaurant just down the bluff from the hotel where we all overate (lamb shank with couscous) and drank too much wine on the terrace watching the sunset.

><

I dialed into the American news as I was curious to see what had happened with the DC rally in support of those arrested for the January 6th riot at the capitol. It looks from the coverage I've seen that it was a complete fizzle with more security present than protesters.

I'm wondering if the MAGA movement is beginning to lose steam, what with its leader out of power, sane adults in power helping keep the economy on track, and finally an awakening that being a contrarian in the face of a deadly virus may not be the best strategy for one's health.

I don't think it's gone by any stretch of the imagination. It will only take the right cultural fertilizer to have it blossom in some new malignant direction. Those sorts of anti-establishment feelings are as old as the country. They need to be acknowledged and their energies channeled in ways that can benefit rather than destroy.

As a physician, the thing I worry about most is what happens when the next pandemic hits. Pandemics are the easiest of natural disasters to predict. They have always happened and always will. We can accept that inevitable truth or ignore it at our peril.

We got away relatively easily with this one as, to date, it has only killed about 0.2% of the population. What happens when the next one comes a decade from now or two decades from now and has a mortality rate of 5% or 10% or 20%? The rancorous distrust of the government, basic public health precepts, the medical system, and medical science that has now become firmly rooted in the culture will hamper our ability to deal at that time in new and unknowable ways.

I worry greatly that COVID, as bad as it has been, is not going to be the real problem. The next pandemic, a more serious disease still, hitting a rickety healthcare system, and a population primed for rejecting the most basic of precautions, is more of a worry.

Here in Spain, with vaccination rates now over 75% and case rates falling, the rules are changing.

Masking is no longer required outdoors in any circumstance, although most people do it in crowd situations as a courtesy. Masking is still universal indoors unless eating or drinking, and the climate is such that most of our meals have actually been outside. I feel perfectly safe moving around the country.

I'm not sure I'll feel as safe back home next week.

Our local bell-weather school system, where the parents fought back against a "conservative" school board and got them to require masking, has noted a significant drop in cases over the last few weeks since masks went into effect. So, of course, they're lifting the mask rule now. Cases to spike up again in 3… 2… 1… And the parent groups, full of physicians and university professors, are marching on the school board again.

But that's not my problem today. My only issue is getting a decent night's sleep before exploring Granada tomorrow.

SUNDAY | SEPTEMBER 19, 2021

GRANADA, NESTLED IN A MOUNTAIN VALLEY near the Sierra Nevada range, was deliciously cool this morning as the mountain winds descended overnight. I actually needed a pullover for the first time this trip. It rapidly warmed up and was in the 80s by noon, but without the humidity of the coastal areas.

Our guide met us this morning and we headed off to the Alham-

341

bra. One of the nice things about Tauck Tours is that they arrange everything in advance so there is no waiting in line. The Alhambra is one of the most visited sites in Europe and access is strictly limited to keep the flow of visitors down to protect 13th- and 14th-century buildings and interiors.

Tickets often have to be reserved months in advance. However, by whatever magic, we were able to walk right in through the magnificent gate of justice and spend the next two and a half hours in the halls, courts, and gardens of the sultans of Granada, the last of the Muslim kingdoms on the Iberian peninsula, lasting from the mid-1200s, after the fall of Seville to the Christians, through a negotiated settlement and withdrawal to Ferdinand and Isabella in 1492.

The fortified palace the Sultans built for themselves on the crest of the hill with its intricate Islamic decorations, beautiful hydraulically engineered fountains (still using the original plumbing system), and acres of courtyard and terraced gardens, was never attacked in war.

Napoleon, on leaving the city late in the Peninsular wars, ordered that it be blown up to deprive the Spanish of a stronghold. But the French were only able to damage the east end of the complex due to some enterprising Spanish soldiers who cut the fuses to the munitions placed in the west end.

It's a sight that must be seen and that I cannot adequately describe. Washington Irving did in the early 19th century in his Tales from the Alhambra, the literary work that put Granada on the cultural map after some years as a backwater.

I haven't read it (or much other Irving except The Legend of Sleepy Hollow and Rip Van Winkle), so I'll have to take our guide's word for it that he got it right, even though apparently the majority of his tales were pure fantasy with no historical truth behind them. I'll settle for the fact that some of the Dorne sequences from Game of Thrones were shot there.

What I've learned from this trip is how little I know about Portuguese/Spanish history. I know some of the general outlines and a few dates but that's about it. American World History tends to focus much more on the British and the French. I'll have to do some reading.

After the tour, we took a walk down the hill through a woodland park to the center of Granada proper. Most of the downtown area is late 19th-century neo-Renaissance of no particular distinction, but coming off of the central commercial district are older residential neighborhoods dating back to Moorish times that could easily be in Marrakesh. Whitewashed walls, a rabbit warren of narrow streets and alleys, little interlinked shops in the manner of an Arab bazaar filled with cheap stuff that seems mainly imported from India. (I did not purchase.)

The cathedral is an amalgam of gothic, renaissance, and baroque built smack in the middle of a residential/commercial district and without a surrounding plaza, making it very difficult to get back from it to get a good look. There were a number of other interesting old churches, a few converted mosques from pre-1492.

A few hours of wandering was enough. I took a taxi back up the hill, so I wouldn't have to climb. My nearly 60-year-old knees are noticing the amount of walking I've been doing. A brief nap and then dinner and a show at the hotel. Dinner—a spicy pork roast. The show—a small revue of traditional flamenco music and dance styles. It was well done, but I couldn't help but think of Ya-Ya in *Strictly Ballroom* saying "You dance the Paso Doble?"

~⊷

COVID news of the day.

The FDA has made its rulings on booster shots clear: if you've had either Pfizer or Moderna, and you are either over 65 or have some sort of immune compromise, get a booster. If you don't fall into those categories, you don't need to. Of course, getting a booster won't hurt you. There just isn't good science that it's of enough benefit to justify a recommendation.

Those who got J-and-J are in limbo. The science regarding boosters just hasn't been done with the same rigor as with the first two, so there are a lot of unknowns. There are no formal recommendations yet. However, a booster, either of J-and-J or of either of the other two, again, is likely not to hurt and may be of some benefit, at least of more benefit than gargling Betadine.

Alabama case counts are down, but the death rate is going up—plus 175% over the last two weeks.

This is right on schedule. Remember that cases spike first, hospitalizations spike two or three weeks after cases, and deaths spike two or three weeks after hospitalizations. The big increase was through the month of August, so mid-September is exactly when we should begin seeing mortality statistics increase.

I can't help but feel sorry for the survivors of the recently deceased. Knowing a thing or two about grief and how it changes your world, there are a lot of people in for some very rough times over the next few years, and it's unnecessary.

Meanwhile, here in Spain, case counts continue to fall, vaccinations continue to rise, and people don't fuss about having to prove vaccination status or wearing masks. I'm going to miss that attitude when I return home next week.

We're up early tomorrow and on to Cordoba. I promise to wash my hands, wear my mask as needed, and keep my distance as much as possible.

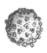

MONDAY | SEPTEMBER 20, 2021

AND ON TO THE LAST LEG OF THE TOUR.

The intrepid eleven—twelve if you include Fernando, our guide, font of all knowledge, translator, and general herder of squirrels, or thirteen if you add in Armenio, our stoic Portuguese bus driver—headed out of Granada as the sun rose. Spain is in the same time zone as France and Germany, but it lies significantly farther west which makes the sun come up late as it should be at least an hour earlier.

After battling rush hour traffic in the suburbs, we entered hill country, marked mainly by commercial olive groves of gray-green trees with the occasional small town in the distance. The towns all look about the same. Whitewashed houses clinging to the side of a hill with a church and citadel on top, the citadel usually in a state of some dis-repair as castles haven't been terribly useful since gunpowder came on the scene in the 16th century. According to Fernando, there are more than 2,000 castles in Spain, most of them in various states of decay.

After a couple of hours, we arrived in Cordoba and were dropped near the old city. Armenio and the bus kept heading toward Madrid with the luggage while we had several hours to explore the town.

Cordoba was a Roman town back in the day and, under the height of the Moorish occupation in the 10th and 11th centuries, was the largest city in Europe with a population in excess of a million while London and Paris had fewer than 20,000 apiece. Its wealth was fueled by its prominence as a river port, complete with Roman bridge across the Guadalquivir, and from nearby gold and silver mines.

The Sultans built an enormous mosque on the banks of the river, enlarged it multiple times, and, when the Christians reconquered the city, rather than raze it as happened in most other Spanish towns, they kept it intact and converted it into a cathedral. Over the years, side chapels were added, and eventually, during the renaissance, a complete Latin cross nave, apse, and transepts were plunked down right in the middle of the building.

The end result, the mosque-cathedral, is highly unusual with elements from Arabic/Byzantine all the way through Baroque in the same building, but it kind of works in an endearing way. The old town is similar to Granada—a maze of twisting alleyways with houses abutting the street, opening into interior courtyards with fountains and flowers. Then it was on to the train to Madrid, a non-stop express of less than two hours.

We arrived just after the bus and luggage and checked into the Palace Hotel, just off the main boulevard, across the street from the parliament building on one side and the Prado museum on the other. It was nearly 6 PM when I got settled, and dinner was at 7:30—not much time to explore—so I walked around the immediate neighborhood and ended up at the Reina Sofia museum, home of Picasso's masterpiece, Guernica. Admission is free after 6 PM. (Score!) And in I went.

I've seen the painting reproduced many times over the years but nothing quite prepared me for the monumental size of the canvas as large as a wall. It's displayed in the midst of a series of galleries that puts it in context, both historic and artistic, which makes it even more powerful.

Paintings from what I suppose is the Spanish equivalent of the Ashcan School of the early 20th century, depict the brutal conditions of urban life and factory work. The explosion of new ideas in the years leading up to and following World War I: Cubism, Surrealism, Dadaism; galleries of how art was used as propaganda including posters and magazine covers; galleries devoted to the decadence of between-the-wars society including a whole lot of Grosz and loops of Bunel film clips.

As I was passing through these, the parallels between those times of wrenching change and our own came leaping off the walls. By the time I got to the Guernica canvas itself, I was in a heightened emotional state. I had to walk around a couple of blocks afterward to maintain my equipoise.

Dinner, in the gorgeous hotel rotunda, was a bit unnerving thereafter—a "pleasures of the bourgeoisie built on the backs of the suffering of the proletariat" moment. I had one more glass of wine than usual and toddled off to my room to ruminate.

I'm sure there's some sort of grand meditation on the nature of society, my place in the world, and how life works germinating in my brain, but I'm not sure tonight's the night to get it out. It's been a long day. I'm going to settle into mindless TV dubbed into some language I don't speak very well.

As one does.

TUESDAY | SEPTEMBER 21, 2021

TODAY WAS OUR FULL DAY IN MADRID.

It's a large city of roughly four million people, but the historic center where most of the interesting sights are located is much smaller and easily walkable.

Cities have always been constrained by time. Inhabitants don't want to spend more than 90 minutes a day commuting, no matter the technology. When transportation was mainly on foot, cities could be crossed in 30-45 minutes and were limited to about four square miles.

The horse and carriage opened that up some. In the 19th century, the invention of the streetcar and public transportation allowed things to expand greatly. And then, finally, the private automobile took over in the mid-20th century, resulting in the endless sprawl of suburbia.

Space is more of an issue in Europe than in America, but even European cities have their modern highrise districts, usually a ways from the historical center, as well as their far-flung suburbs, usually small outlying towns incorporated into burgeoning metro areas.

I have always loved visiting the historic centers of European cities. They are designed around the pedestrian with cars as an afterthought. I have always enjoyed just walking. (My pedometer is very happy with me this trip. I'm averaging 16,000–20,000 steps a day.)

On my first trip to Europe, when I was 22, I crammed as much into eight weeks as I could, often sleeping on the train overnight between destinations and then covering things on foot at a brisk clip.

My knees, however, are no longer in their early 20s and are complaining a bit as we approach the two-week mark, but I only have a couple of days to go. They'll make it with the help of some Arthritis-strength Tylenol. I just have to keep reminding myself that 22 was nearly four decades ago.

Most American cities were laid out later in historical development than European ones so they aren't walkable in the same way. They came to be after public transportation or the car were well established and took primacy. Few are truly walkable. I treasure the exceptions: Boston, New York, San Francisco, New Orleans.

The first part of the day was a bus tour of the city including some of the outlying districts. It's my least favorite way to see a city and I can't say I enjoyed it much, but it gave me a chance to get oriented.

After an hour, we ended up at the Prado Art Museum, one of the few great museums of Western Art that I had not previously visited. It features multiple masterpieces of the great Spanish painters—Velasquez, Murillo, Goya, El Greco; some decent Italian post-Renaissance art commissioned when Spain was the richest country in Europe during the late 16th and early 17th centuries; also some interesting Dutch pieces as Spain owned the Low Countries in the post-Renaissance period including most of the masterworks of Bosch. It was great fun to finally see *The Garden of Earthly Delights* in the flesh for the first time. I have long been familiar with it, having had a poster of it up in my college freshman dorm room, as one does.

After the Prado, Fernando, our fearless leader, who lives in Madrid, gave us a walking backstreet tour of his favorite haunts. This was much more to my taste than the bus ride as I was able to get more of a feel of the look and the rhythms of the city when not seated at a height, sealed away by air conditioning and glass.

We ended up back at the hotel where I got a brain biopsy of a COVID test so I can fly back to the US in a couple of days (negative again). Then we were on our own until morning.

I used my time to do a little shopping, to wander some backstreets in more usual residential areas, and to have dinner and a margarita in a little hole in the wall that turned out to have excellent food.

We've got one more tour day, tomorrow, and then, on Thursday, I have to surface back into reality. I was supposed to stay in Madrid until Sunday, but I canceled the extra days so I would be under the care of the tour operators regarding COVID testing and flights home.

After logging in something over 24,000 steps today on the pedometer, my legs are tired. I have returned to my room early so I can be refreshed for the trip to Toledo in the morning.

＞◦＜

There have been a bunch of COVID vaccine headlines over the last couple of days. I don't have complete information but here are my two big takeaways.

349

1. Kids

Pfizer has released study data showing its vaccine is safe and effective down to five years of age. This is drug company data that has not yet been vetted by the FDA, so don't bother your pediatrician for shots yet. If the data is as clean as it appears to be, the FDA will approve shots for children 5-11 in a couple of months, at least on an Emergency Use Authorization.

Moderna hasn't released its data yet, but it is likely to be similar. I haven't seen anything about J-and-J for kids, but I'm sure it's being studied.

2. Boosters

Get one if you're immuno-compromised in any way or if you're over 65. While it's recommended you remain on the same team, it probably doesn't hurt to switch hit.

J-and-J released data today showing that a booster of their formulation is helpful, but there are no formal instructions yet as we are, again, still dealing with drug company data. (I have learned over the years to take drug company data and press releases with a very large grain of salt).

We have officially passed the 1918-19 flu pandemic in terms of the number of deaths. COVID is now the greatest mass casualty event in the history of the US with fatalities of 675,000 and climbing. The Delta spike will continue to add to the toll at a rapid pace over the next couple of months, then there may be a lull.

It's hard to predict.

There could be a new variant with significantly higher transmission or mortality. We could have a new outbreak of politically fueled negative behaviors. A variant could outsmart the vaccine.

Then there's the question of Africa: a continent of poor countries that has had little luck getting any vaccine whatsoever for its populace, leaving a huge potential population in which trouble could lurk.

We tend to forget that a pandemic is global and, for it to be brought under control, global solutions are required. This means more than just the wealthy countries of the world taking care of themselves.

Tired now. Must get some sleep.

WEDNESDAY | SEPTEMBER 22, 2021

TODAY IS THE LAST DAY OF THE TOUR; there's just one more destination to hit: Toledo.

Madrid is the current capital city, but the capital was only moved here in the 17th century. The Hapsburgs and the Bourbons needed more room for palaces and additional population. Toledo, the capital since the Visigoths occupied Iberia during the collapse of the Roman Empire, was left in the dust.

Toledo is an hour away by train, car, or bus, an easy jaunt first thing in the morning. We had a few brief showers on the trip and the skies were glowering when we got there, but things brightened up through the morning and our luck with the weather continued.

As the medieval capital, Toledo is very much still a medieval town. Built on a high bluff where the River Tagus makes a large oxbow bend through a gorge, it was easily defensible as a walled city. It's also easy to see why the kings scampered after the introduction of gunpowder into warfare that made such fortifications obsolete.

The city retains a true Middle Ages feel: winding narrow lanes with no rhyme or reason; fortified buildings, some dating back nearly a thousand years; it has a sense of unreality to it as if it's some sort of movie set or theme park. If you go around the next corner, you may stumble into Adventureland.

The approach to the city, by a winding road on the opposite side of the gorge, lays it out before you, looking like one of the city sets from *Game of Thrones*. I half expected the Alcazar or the Cathedral to suddenly start unfolding as a little mechanical toy.

We toured the city on foot; my favorite way to do things. The highlight was the cathedral: Spanish Gothic with a great altarpiece and a stunning collection of El Greco paintings. (He was based in Toledo most of his working life). I've always liked his work. It's incredibly modern looking for a Renaissance master.

I'm not sure about the Baroque addition in the apse, a dome and rococo fantasia of a back altar constructed several hundred years after the original building was finished in order to let in more light. We made a few other stops including a chapel where we saw a massive El Greco, as well as the original synagogue from the 11th century, built for the Jews by the Moors and looking all the world like a mosque.

We lunched at a hacienda snuggled up on the town walls: roast suckling pig and several other courses. Then our busload of napping and sated tourists headed back to Madrid.

I did a last-minute shop-and-wander, and then returned for the second gala meal of the day (not having fully digested the first): a farewell dinner (sea bass) accompanied by several wines and champagne.

Dinner entertainment was provided by a rather good quartet of Spanish guitarists/mandolin players/vocalists doing the few songs in Spanish that American tourists tend to know: *Guantanamera, Malaguena, Granada, Besame Mucho,* etc.

To accompany dessert, the assembled crew demanded that I entertain them with something. I was just tiddly enough to do it, so I found a karaoke track on YouTube on my phone and gave them a rousing edition of *Don't Tell Mama*. (I figured I had to do something unexpected.) Hopefully, no one recorded it.

Now to bed and then the return home through three airports and two airplanes tomorrow. I have my passport, my ticket, my negative COVID test. I figure the US will let me back in.

Keep your hands and noses clean, and wear your masks indoors. Spain is lifting more and more restrictions as no one is dying over here and most of the population is vaccinated. They may be back to normal in the new year.

I wonder where we'll be?

SATURDAY | SEPTEMBER 25, 2021

'M STARTING TO SURFACE FOR AIR after a couple of days of torpor.

The flights on my protracted trip back home from Spain were uneventful. Just a lot of hurry up and wait as one usually gets these days with air travel.

Air traffic appears to be picking back up. It's nowhere as crazy as it was pre-COVID, but both the Madrid and the Atlanta airports were more full than they were on my outbound journey not quite three weeks ago.

There were no episodes of air rage or bad behavior on my flights. It may become more frequent as mental health, in general, deterio-rates and the pandemic grinds on, but if the airlines start sharing their no-fly lists with each other, and people start to find themselves barred from all air travel if they don't act like adults rather than toddlers in a snit, this particular facet of modern life will likely take care of itself.

The only hitch in the return trip was the complete dearth of ground transportation when I landed in Birmingham. Attendees at the Furnace Fest music festival had apparently commandeered every taxi, Uber, and Lyft in the metro area on Thursday. Fortunately, I have phone-a-friend capabilities.

><===

The weather has broken, the humidity is gone, and the tang of fall is in the air. We're getting into my favorite time of year.

I've always been an autumn person. Fall to me means new beginnings and gearing up for new possibilities as I have been tied to the American academic calendar since age five.

Growing up, fall also meant the glorious Indian Summer days of a Seattle September, sunny without being warm, leaves beginning to change, and a prolonged magic hour in the late afternoon with a golden light from the setting sun so thick you could almost cut it with a knife. I've never seen anything quite like it anywhere else I have lived. Must have something to do with the latitude.

Fall also means a chill in the air at night, so I've flipped the HVAC from cool to heat. The cats, who went into hiding for the first twelve hours or so after my arrival, have decided I'm me, have reemerged, and are going about their usual routines. I've done the laundry and the grocery shopping, unpacked, and, in general, started the process of getting back to normal life.

><===

The number of COVID inpatients at UAB has been steadily declining. Hopefully, that means that the worst of the Delta surge locally is over and things will calm down a bit and let everyone take a breather. However, the death rate is skyrocketing (as it does about four to six weeks after a surge begins). Alabama's death rate per population is currently the highest in the country, about double that of every other state.

We had 123 deaths yesterday. Our 7-day average is 125 a day. By comparison, Spain, where I just was, had 44 deaths yesterday with a seven-day average of 64—*across the entire country.* When you consider that Spain has three-and-a-half-to-four times the population of Alabama, which place is doing a better job keeping its population out of harm's way?

It's been a bit of an adjustment coming back and seeing people serenely waltz in and out of buildings without masks, hearing about local schools lifting mask mandates due to their "conservative values", seeing various snake oil cures (some of which are downright dangerous like nebulizing hydrogen peroxide) being touted as appropriate protocols by people without medical training, and having prominent politicians bragging to the media about how they have spent the last 18 months listening to professional public health advice and then doing the opposite.

Just a few weeks in Spain, a society that understood and accepted basic mitigation measures as necessary for the common good, did them without complaint or fuss, and who got their vaccinations without a major blowback movement, seems to have spoiled me.

The State Department still has Portugal and Spain as Level 4 travel advisories (do not travel there without urgent need due to COVID risk). They've been listed like that since July. It's ridiculous. I feel much more endangered here than I ever did there. (If Spain is Level 4, we should make Alabama Level 5 and Florida Level 6.)

I'm trying to decide what the last few weeks of away time and decompression have meant.

Was it just a chance to get away and see a part of the world I had not yet been to? Was it a time to contrast and compare a society that has done public health basics in a non-political way with our own craziness that seems bound and determined to push the death toll ever higher?

Was it a way to get my head in a different space so I know where and how to point myself next? If it was, it was pretty much a flop; I still haven't figured out what the next chapter of life holds, so I'll more or less return to old patterns until I do.

One thing I did figure out is that I'd like to find a travel companion for my next major jaunt. If you think you're that person, give me a call and we'll discuss it.

I don't have my big 2022 trip set yet. It's going to depend on COVID and work and theater and the writing of books and all the rest of the things that collide on my calendar. I do have a companion set for my trip to London at New Year's, so I'll be able to do some comparing and contrasting with how that works.

MONDAY | SEPTEMBER 27, 2021

I T'S BACK TO THE GRIND TOMORROW.

It's been nice to have been off for a few weeks and had a chance to do some fun things and rest up, but there are people to care for and bills to pay and house calls to make, and all of the other usual chores of my workaday life.

I've been spending this last day making sure I have all of my tasks and deadlines for the next few weeks ready to go. Three lectures to write? Check. A show to audition for? Check. Two book-signing events to plan? Check. Various social invitations responded to and entered into the calendar? Check.

My next-door neighbors are in the process of a major remodel. Usually, this isn't a problem as I'm rarely home during working hours, but today—a day that involved workmen pounding on the shared wall most of the time, when they weren't using power tools with various dissonant pitches—I was getting a little frazzled. At least they knocked off for an hour at lunch when I had a Zoom call—a brief reading and Q-and-A about the book for a local civic group.

I decided to drown out the cacophony from next door with some television turned up high. I put on Apple TV in order to catch up with a couple of streaming series that have made a lot of stir in my social media circles but which I had not yet seen.

The first was *Schmigadoon,* the send-up of the golden age Rodgers and Hammerstein-type American musical. I enjoyed it as I had no problems recognizing all of the tropes—visual, musical, and characterological—that the makers were lampooning.

From the orchestration of the overture (right out of *Oklahoma!)* to deft parodies of Marian Paroo, Og the Leprechaun, Billy Bigelow, and Daisy Mae, I was smiling throughout but was rarely bowled over with laughter.

It was cute and clever, but it was missing the thing that those shows all had: a solid emotional core. *Ya Gotta Have Heart!* And it was missing.

I couldn't figure out at the end who the audience for it was supposed to be. Most people under 50 or 60 wouldn't recognize the references, and the numbers of theater kids and theater queens is quite small when compared to the total population. I guess that's a bonus for this new model of streaming services. The ability to create shows for niche audiences that need not have the best ratings.

I then turned to *Ted Lasso.*

I haven't finished it yet, being only on episode four, but I quite like it. What is amazing to me about the show and the character is that an example of goodness and empathy, which would have been a fairly standard type in the programming of not-so-many years ago is now, in the age of Trump, seen as something of a novelty.

Ted is a fish out of water and not well-spoken. He puts himself in ridiculous situations but is, at his core, such a decent and moral person who sees his mission as helping others become their best selves, that I can't help but root for him.

The joy of the series is watching the transformations in the other characters (surrogates for ourselves and our society) grow and change under his presence. It's the perfect antidote for these Trumpian times, and it's no wonder it cleaned up at the Emmys recently.

Perhaps more flawed, but empathetic and generally good characters will enter our pop culture consciousness and help nudge the pendulum back a little bit from the selfishness and negativity that seem to be the order of the day.

Speaking of selfishness, it's time to return to the COVID wars.

The CDC produced a very sound scientific study of schools yesterday showing that schools with mask mandates were far less likely to have COVID breakouts than those without. It's one of those water-is-wet studies whose conclusions seem relatively obvious, but it's nice to see some science behind the common sense that can be used with recalcitrant school boards who feel that owning the libs is more important than protecting their children.

The current Delta wave is going to create a huge bill to pay in terms of children's issues in the future. The deaths are spiking and many of the dead are relatively young adults between 25 and 50 who are leaving orphaned children behind. I don't know that anyone is tracking the number of minor children who have lost one or both parents to COVID so far, but I'm sure it's in the thousands, if not the tens of thousands.

In the original waves, before vaccination, it was a tragedy but now, with the disease being more or less preventable, at least in its fatal form, these parents are choosing an idea based on fallacies and cynical political opportunism over the love and needs of their own children.

When the kids mature enough to understand that MAGA was more important to their parents than they were, what is that going to do to their mental health and to their understanding of their place in the world?

><>

War and opposing political philosophies have always created orphans, but those sacrifices have usually been made in the name of something positive, something better—a freer society for children, protection of the populace from invasion.

The current conservative philosophy as espoused by those who would deny science and public health doesn't appear to stand for much, at least to me. It's rooted strictly in being in opposition—to progress, to a more equal society, to benefits flowing down the socio-economic ladder rather than up.

This is my major objection to much of the current rhetoric on the right. Tell me what you want for the country and how you want to get there. I'll listen. Throwing a tantrum at every suggestion just makes me want to put you in the corner for a time out.

There seems to be some idea espoused that they want to go back, ostensibly, to the America of *Leave it to Beaver* and *Sally, Dick, and Jane*, a time that never actually existed other than in carefully crafted cultural items designed to lull the developing Baby Boom into a false sense of security.

You can't go back, ever. Time doesn't work that way. You can only go forward.

The only thing that seems to motivate the way forward is en-trenching a minority rule through selective legislation. You may be able to do that in the short run, but it's rarely a successful long-term strategy for societal stability.

If I have to choose between an America as embodied by *Ted Lasso* or an America as embodied by a horde of screaming suburbanites invading the local mall food court because they've been asked to do something as simple as wear a mask, I'll take Ted.

I'll bet he keeps his hands washed, wears his mask, keeps his distance, and got his shots publicly in front of the whole team as an example.

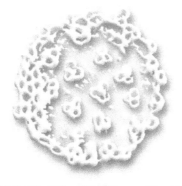

OCTOBER 2021
I've Still Got My Health

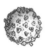

SATURDAY | OCTOBER 2, 2021

7 00,000.

That's the number of American deaths from COVID since the beginning of the pandemic. That's roughly equivalent to the population of Boston or Washington DC. It's also about the same as the number of American deaths from HIV (just a bit over 714,000).

HIV took 40 years to hit that number. COVID has done it in 18 months.

The death toll has been pretty steady over the last week or so as those sickened by the Delta wave in August are in the midst of their inevitable die-off. There are still plenty of critically ill in the hospital.

Even though admission numbers, on the whole, are trending downward, ICU numbers remain shockingly high, and now include mainly previously young and healthy people.

A number of states—Alaska, Idaho, the Dakotas—continue to max out their ability to care for the seriously ill and are working under various sorts of triage and rationing of care. It's just not possible to be all things to all comers in the situation in which we currently find ourselves.

Someone much more intelligent than I once said of health care that it can be inexpensive, it can be universal, and it can be of high quality—but it can only be two of those things at any one time. No one has yet invented a system that delivers all three simultaneously.

At the moment, given the stresses of the coronavirus, our health-care system is having difficulties delivering even one of these things at a time, and I don't foresee things getting better in the near future.

Eighteen months of societal stress, toxic work environments, emphasis on payment over people, bad behavior by the general public, and a host of other factors, large and small, have ground down the human capital of our system.

Nurses are leaving their jobs in droves, some to do other things, some to take advantage of the enormous salaries being offered by temp staffing agencies in providing qualified bodies to desperate hospital systems. I've heard of travel nurses making roughly double what I make with assignments to COVID wards—and I don't begrudge them a penny.

I had my annual review this week with UAB. (Relax, I have a job for another year, my 24th with them). My big comment was this: What is UAB going to do to help me not choose early retirement as my best option in life? Something for both me and my powers that be to think upon.

I did a couple of Zoom book club meetings this week about Volume One of The Accidental Plague Diaries, one with a civic group and one with a UAB audience. The most interesting question posed to me was this: Where do I stand with the idea that the willfully unvaccinated be refused treatment for complications of COVID infection?

That got me thinking about medical ethics and what I truly believe.

Everyone knows about physicians and the Hippocratic oath.

Most US medical schools no longer use it. It's over 2500 years old and has odd things in it that probably made sense to the Ancient Greeks but which don't apply these days such as not having sex with the maids when making a house call. It also prohibits surgery.

At my graduation ceremony from medical school, we used something called The Physician's Oath which is similar in spirit, even if it doesn't have quite the same storied tradition. Med schools these days make a lot more pomp and circumstance about such things than they did back when I was in training.

There is now a "White Coat Ceremony" for entering medical students where they are given their white coats and are sworn to uphold medical ethics. My white coat ceremony was going to the bookstore, grabbing the right size off the rack, and being told 'That'll be $17.95" by a bored cashier.

There is great symbolism in the white coat.

It's the ceremonial robe that reminds everyone that we are descended from the priesthood, interceding with the gods for a favorable outcome in the eternal battle between health and disease. And, just as with priests, there is a sacred bond between the intercessor and he or she who seeks help.

We are told things that people do not share with anyone else. We're regarded as a safe space for the unburdening of feelings, emotions, and unanswerable questions.

In an ideal world, healer and patient form a dyad that together find a path forward. The healer becomes the advocate for the patient on the journey and is answerable to no one and nothing but the needs of the patient. But we don't live in an ideal world.

In the American system, there are multiple layers of entities inserting their tentacles into that bubble. Financial, quality assurance, legal, clerical—the list goes on. It's easy to lose one's way.

It still boils down to the fact that the physician is responsible to the patient—the person sitting in front of him/her at any given time and, ethically, the healer is bound to put the needs of that patient above all other considerations.

Therefore, the willfully unvaccinated are as deserving of treatment as smokers with lung cancer, the overweight with diabetes, and rock climbers with broken arms. We can't make judgment calls on the circumstances that bring patients to us; we only look forward, not back.

The argument then becomes, what about the costs to society of these choices?

Society has every right to impose whatever rules it sees fit with regard to these costs. This could include surcharges on insurance, requirements for vaccination to continue employment, etc. But these are not rules for a physician to employ within the dyad of care.

If you're my patient, I will do whatever I think is necessary to get you the treatment I think you need to restore your health and function. I may run into brick walls imposed by the system or by society at large, but then it becomes my job to try to find a way over or under or around if I can. Sometimes I win, sometimes I don't, but I have to try.

I suppose this particular tilting at windmills is what gives me my love for Don Quixote. My gift to myself from my recent vacation is a hand-painted tile of him and Sancho Panza.

The costs to society run up by the willfully unvaccinated are now in the billions of dollars: money spent on acute care hospitalization, money needed to care for orphaned children, money to help support those who have survived but who are not healthy enough to return to their previous lives.

Society will continue to react to this. Some of this reaction will manifest through the legal system as new laws and rules, but most of it, I think, will come through the economic system as corporate interests of various stripes seek to shield themselves from losses and liabilities.

Where and how will it end? And what will things look like six months or a year from now? I don't know, but I imagine it's going to be harder and harder for the willfully unvaccinated to access public transportation or venues of public accommodation.

I read somewhere that a significant portion of these individuals would like to secede from the country. I wonder how their utopia would fare in a globalized world and economy without continued support from urban and coastal America? I imagine it would devolve into something akin to one of the poorer countries of sub-Saharan Africa within a decade.

It's Saturday night.

I should be out tripping the light fantastic somewhere, but I'd rather stay curled up with the cats (one of whom leapt up on the dinner table, started lapping up my ranch dressing, and had to be whacked on the butt), and a nice bottle of red wine.

Be safe, be well, wash your hands, get your vaccines.

WEDNESDAY | OCTOBER 6, 2021

THE HEADLINES TODAY were about the total number of COVID deaths in 2021 exceeding the total number in 2020. It's not a totally fair comparison.

COVID didn't take hold in the US until March 2020. It didn't begin to cause significant mortality until April 2020. For statistical purposes, 2020 was only nine months long. We're now in early October, just over nine months into 2021 when we hit the equivalency mark, so we're actually at roughly the same place.

The issue, of course, is that with our continued high levels of willfully unvaccinated individuals, we're likely to see much higher levels of mortality continuing over the remaining three months of 2021 than we did in the last quarter of 2020. Will we see the same kind of numbers in 2022? Time will tell.

We're on the downside of the Delta wave here in the Deep South. Hospital censuses are declining and new diagnoses are fewer.

Why is the wave receding? Hard to say. It's likely multifactorial.

It may involve slight changes in public behavior and group inter-action as the wave was intensifying in August. Small increases in vac-cination rates might have large ripple effects. There may be climatic issues at work.

With luck, we've seen the worst of it for a while. However, human behavior being what it is, a general relaxation of masks and social dis-tancing may lead to numbers going back up again as we start crowd-ing indoors in colder weather.

Things are certainly not improving yet in the Mountain West and in Alaska where the hospitals are past the breaking point and various triage measures have been put in place to protect scarce resources.

Should there be national standards for such things?

Americans are loathe to deny anyone anything once they become patients in the healthcare industry. For 40 years now, I've observed what I call pit bull medicine. The system will sink its teeth into cer-tain complex critically ill individuals, hang on for dear life, and shake them until death or payments stop, whichever comes first.

This is less common now than it was several decades ago with the rise of palliative care, hospice programs, and other more humane ways of dealing with the human condition, but it hasn't been com-pletely eliminated. When looking around at various regional differ-ences, I've always found it most prevalent in Florida. This is one of the reasons I took the job here in Alabama over several possibilities in that state back when I relocated.

And now, a somewhat related story about relatively recent medical history.

In the not too distant past, kidney failure was a death sentence. There was nothing that could be done for someone who had non-functional organs charged with processing and removing the toxic byproducts of metabolism. These compounds would accumulate and their poisonous effects would eventually overwhelm the body.

In the mid-1970s, researchers at the University of Washington invented the first practical hemodialysis machines. Word got around about this wondrous new technology and every nephrologist was eager to have their patients selected for this life-saving intervention. It was still experimental and there wasn't money to produce dialysis machines in quantity, so the slots available for patients were limited. How to decide who would live and who would not?

A committee was formed. Its membership was (and remains to this day) secret.

It included physicians, ethicists, clergy, patient representatives, etc. It was soon dubbed the *God Committee* as patients would make applications for dialysis and, based on their rankings, some received it and some did not.

The federal government got wind of the concept and was upset about the idea of Americans sitting in life and death judgment over other Americans. What to do?

The solution was money.

Legislation was passed to make the diagnosis of End-Stage Renal Disease requiring dialysis an automatic qualification for Medicare and, with a steady stream of revenue now in place, more and more machines could be built. In short order, anyone who needed dialysis could get it.

The downside of this is that the profit motive has led to any number of people who other health systems would consider unsuitable candidates for a medical procedure (comatose, end-stage dementia, etc.) to be regularly dialyzed in the American system as there's money to be made.

I advise my patients in their 80s and above to think long and hard about committing to dialysis. It's rough on the body, rough on lifestyles, and rough on families. It's ultimately not my choice, but theirs, and I will support them in whatever they choose. Those who do not choose it, but who will pay attention to diet, fluid balance, and the like, will often fare just as well and live just as long as those who do.

The elder body can often adapt in spectacular ways if you let it. It doesn't take that many nephrons to keep it going. Doing this sort of counseling, of course, takes time, good rapport, and a knowledge of one's patients as individuals. Learning who my patients are and coming to understand their stories are what keep me interested in my professional life.

✄◄═

One of my rural house call patients died this past week.

He was 94, so it wasn't unexpected, but he had been in quite reasonable shape. He had a sudden cardiac decompensation at home and died within 48 hours at the local hospital. He didn't suffer unduly, and he had been independent up until his final illness.

He was a long-time widower without children who lived in a small house in Jasper. He had a younger brother who would check up on him once a week or so. His next-door neighbors were friendly and helped him out when they could.

He was quiet and unassuming. We admitted him to the VA house call program about three years ago after a bad fall onto concrete in his carport which served as a wake-up call that he needed a little more monitoring than he could give himself.

He was a World War II Vet. He joined the Navy in the waning days of the war. On V-J Day, he was in Times Square, 18 years old, dressed in his ill-fitting sailor's whites, walking through the crowd and, through serendipity, he walked into immortality.

Photographer Alfred Eisenstaedt, taking pictures of the revelry, snapped a photo of a kiss that afternoon that became one of the most iconic images of 20th century America, and my patient unknowingly was part of it. His goofy grin as he looked at the couple helped make the picture what it was and still is.

Rest well Mr. Hicks, I salute you.

MONDAY | OCTOBER 11, 2021

THOUGHT TONIGHT I'd take a look at why anti-vaccination is such a big thing.

There's nothing new about the willful flouting of public health dicta by certain segments of American society. There's a strong independent streak in the national character that flows out of the individualism of Western philosophical thought and the Enlightenment: the idea that the individual is the natural building block of society and that each unique individual is to be celebrated for his or her differences is central to our governance, our economy, and our sense of self-understanding.

A couple of other fundamental precepts come with this. One is the idea of bodily autonomy. That our bodies belong wholly and totally to ourselves and that no one has the right to tell us what to do with them against our conscience. Of course, we have all sorts of laws and customs that subvert this. Technically, our bodies no longer belong to ourselves or our heirs after our death.

For reasons of public health, laws exist in every state making the body technically property of the state so that the state can proscribe what can and cannot be done with it postmortem. For example, you're not allowed to plant your mother under your geraniums or expose your hated brother-in-law on the wheel for the elements and the neighbors to gawk at—even though these would have been considered perfectly normal behaviors in times past.

Then there's the penal system under whose care bodily autonomy is strongly limited. There are laws limiting reproductive capability. Rules regarding sexual mores based on consanguinity and chronological age and, of course, all the political thought of the social contract that your rights stop when your actions impinge on my rights.

But this idea, which is basic to medical ethics, is what allows a Jehovah's Witness to refuse blood products, prevents agents of the state from forcing us to donate blood or tissue, or lets us forgo aggressive care at the end of life with a Do Not Resuscitate order.

This also makes it easy for competent adults to refuse a vaccine that would benefit themselves and society as a whole. They need not have any reason for it beyond a simple declaration of "No."

Then, of course, there's the idea that if we are all different, there must be ways of ordering us and, given the way humans categorize and find patterns, even in randomness, there must be a hierarchy among humans—with some of greater and some of lesser worth.

Vaccine mandates and vaccine refusal are as old as the country.

In the early 18th century, a West African slave of Cotton Mather, Onsemus, introduced Mather to a traditional practice of his tribe. They would inoculate themselves with small doses of smallpox to build immunity to the disease. When a smallpox outbreak hit Boston in 1721, Cotton Mather convinced Boston physicians to try the technique.

Records from the time showed that the mortality rate in the inoculated population was 2% compared to 15% in uninoculated individuals. There was some push for more widespread use of the technique, but a number of newspapers were critical, including the newspaper run by the brothers Franklin—James and Benjamin.

Some years later, in 1736, after Benjamin had relocated to Philadelphia, there was a smallpox outbreak in that city, and Ben refused to allow his family to be inoculated. His four-year-old son caught the disease and died. Franklin quickly shifted his position to pro-inoculation and deeply regretted the decision that cost his son his life.

In 1777, George Washington mandated smallpox inoculation for the Continental Army as he was losing more troops to disease than to battle. I'm sure there was some negative reaction to this decision, but as it was a time of war with very real consequences should the war be lost, reactions were muted and were not made much of by the writers of the day.

All of this, of course, took place in a very different society.

Pandemic illness and death were part of the natural order. Everyone saw young healthy people sicken and die from diseases that would easily be cured today such as an infected wound or pneumonia. Young women died of complications in childbirth. Men died young in agricultural or industrial accidents. From early childhood, people grew to understand that the world could be a dark and dangerous place and that simple misadventure could be fatal.

For modern generations, raised in a world of antibiotics, globalism, all-volunteer military, and innumerable workplace safety standards, bad has been safely removed from most of our lives for decades. When pandemic illness struck this past year, as it always has, it struck a population with a lack of coping mechanisms and understanding about the nature of illness and death.

It's not something that happens to people like them, so they need not take it seriously. They need not toe the line regarding public health rules. They can safely question expertise from the cocoon of their own thinking and develop their own alternative theories given their ability to access vast quantities of information via the Internet— although they may not understand or interpret what they find correctly. Alexander Pope put it best when he wrote that "A little learning is a dangerous thing."

Humans, when confronted with realities that do not conform to their expectations or experience, tend to develop elaborate rationalizations and alternatives that fit comfortably within their worldview.

I went to a play this weekend, a one-woman monologue based on Joan Didion's books chronicling her personal experiences with illness, grief, and loss. She entitled her work *The Year of Magical Thinking* in which she attempts to explain her lack of rationality at the sudden death of her husband and the serious illness of her daughter, both of which hit her life nearly simultaneously.

I had read the book some years ago. It was a favorite of Tommy's. He had seen the play in New York with Vanessa Redgrave. The material really spoke to him.

Tommy's early adult life coincided with the first wave of the HIV epidemic. He was deeply involved in the Birmingham gay community's mobilization to face both the needs of the sufferers and the indifference of the general populace.

I can't remember why I didn't go to the play with him. I think it was on a trip he made to New York on his own for some reason, or maybe it was one we made together and I had a meeting or something I had to go to that afternoon. It all escapes me now.

Anyway, as I was watching the performance, I could not help but draw parallels between the magical thinking of Joan Didion in the face of great calamity and the magical thinking of segments of American society when it comes to pandemic response—in particular, the jettisoning of hundreds of years of carefully gathered data and medical facts which tell us how to respond to pandemic disease in favor of praying for divine intervention or trusting the quick cures of charlatans.

Social media has certainly played a role in the spread of fringe ideas.

I regard social media as a tool and, like any tool, it can be used either constructively or destructively. A hammer has no moral value in and of itself. It can be wielded with careful intent to help create something lasting and beautiful, or it can just as easily be used in a malicious fashion to maim or to kill.

Facebook is the same way. You can use it to connect and build community and share positive things, or you can use it to argue and sow divisiveness and discord.

One of the great appeals of social media is its ability to allow isolated members of outcast and minority groups to find each other, create community, and build a social infrastructure. This can be a positive and comforting thing, but it also means that all kinds of communities can coalesce, including some whose purpose is spreading a gospel far outside of usual mainstream thought.

Social media provides a platform and a megaphone for eccentric notions, making it possible for ideas that would once have never made it past a couple of people exchanging letters to infiltrate large groups and begin changing the terms of public discourse.

Once an idea is out there in the zeitgeist, the famed Overton window can start shifting, both left and right, making it harder and harder for society to find the common ground in the middle and the compromise that's necessary for civil social function

We're certainly seeing this in our politics. The result is a Congress that can barely pass legislation and is no longer attending to the business of the general public.

Elected officials, of course, are no longer responsive to their constituents, especially on the national level. They are responsive to those who fund their increasingly expensive re-election campaigns. The general public, of course, does not have the resources to set up PACs and funnel multi-millions to campaign coffers, so politicians now cater to the large corporations and the wealthy individuals who do.

The general tilt of these funders is toward the protection of their perquisites and assets, so legislation such as tax cuts becomes more popular than legislation that might benefit the majority of the citizenry. The upper-middle and professional classes have been co-opted into supporting this agenda by the replacement of the traditional defined benefit pension plan with the IRA and the 401K.

This particular sleight of hand has millions of voters supporting an economic agenda that's better for the stock market, in which their future is heavily invested, rather than one which might, over time, provide them with more tangible benefits in terms of more robust social and health programs.

The conflicts in society that this has put in place have been good for business. Conflict stokes fear and anger and keeps people tuning in to media, clicking on web links, buying books with political themes, and loading themselves up with merchandise that identifies them as Team Red or Team Blue.

Politics has moved from a realm of serious thinkers and policy wonks to just another field of celebrity infotainment where elected officials jockey with each other for camera time or press mentions, adhering to the age-old idea of there's no such thing as bad publicity.

A political system that is no longer terribly interested in the people's business leaves a vacuum for other interests to move in and take care of things that need to be seen to. These are often economic in nature and this has certainly applied to the American healthcare system.

I have written at length in the past about the morphing of our healthcare system into a healthcare industry over the last half-century with a completely new set of rules guiding how it works, not rules pertaining to the saving of lives and general health of the citizenry, but rules ensuring that profit is generated and flows upwards to the owners of the various components of the industry.

Most Americans are fairly happy with their doctors and other healthcare providers on a one-on-one basis. We're well educated, we try to uphold our oaths to our patients and profession, and, in general, we are reasonable communicators.

At the same time, most Americans recognize that the healthcare system is no longer serving them the way it once did.

Their doctors are all of a sudden "out of network." They receive enormous surprise bills for simple emergency visits. They feel like they have very little control over the shape of their healthcare once they enter a hospital.

All of this has fed a distrust of the system, in general, and has helped undermine confidence in medical expertise, in particular, especially when it's coming from "the system" rather than from an individual provider with whom a relationship has been built.

Add to this the systemic racism of American society which manifests itself in healthcare as it does elsewhere—(not to mention such things as the Tuskegee experiments which occurred within living memory, not ending until 1972); the unfamiliarity of most providers, who come from middle and upper-middle-class backgrounds, with the realities of life on the lower end of the socio-economic scale; and the tendency for more and more health care to be handled algorithmically rather than individually—and you get a perfect storm for a patient base to become alienated from the system that's supposed to care for it.

When you start putting all of this together, you start to see that a reaction against public health measures and vaccine mandates was probably inevitable and that the issue is not that we as Americans don't want to be safe from pandemic disease but that we have built social structures over the last half-century that make it nigh on impossible for us to be safe from pandemic disease.

Can this be fixed?

It's not going to be easy. It's going to take a lot of work. It's going to take unified messages from government and media sources which means eliminating the dichotomies and conflicts on which so much of the marketplace is based, potentially reducing profits.

It's going to require Americans having access to health care in a form that they recognize provided by individuals with whom they can form relationships and develop trust, meaning we're going to have to shift the system from one that rewards specialty care to one that rewards primary care.

It's going to require schools that teach critical thinking and how to analyze presented information to understand what it is, what it says, and what the motivations are of the source which presents it, not schools that are focused on teaching to a standardized test. It won't be easy, but nothing worth achieving ever is.

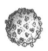

FRIDAY | OCTOBER 15, 2021

I HAD A SPEAKING GIG THIS AFTERNOON.

It was an hour on gero-pharmacy, one of the topics I tackle fairly routinely. It's an important one for anyone involved in the area of elder health to be somewhat conversant with.

I covered things like changing physiology, adverse drug reactions, and adherence strategies—the usual things. It was still a hard gig to do. It hadn't occurred to me when I agreed to do it that the venue, Canterbury United Methodist Church, had some loaded associations for me.

When I've spoken there in the past, it's usually been in their large conference hall, so I assumed this program would be there. It wasn't. It was in their modern worship space—a space I last entered a little over three years ago to attend Tommy's memorial service.

I'm pretty good at turning myself off and doing my job when I need to, so when I started to feel things as I prepared for my talk, I shut them down and got myself ready to do what I was tasked with doing. I gave my talk, I told my jokes, and I put away the part of me that was uncomfortable and emotional until afterward.

When I give lectures, especially on topics I speak about frequently, I have set bits of patter and anecdote to go along with the topic at hand. I don't remember them per se, but when the right slide comes up with the triggering factoid in place, they drop into my brain, I run through the macro, and it's on to the next bit. I have no idea if other people do public speaking this way, but it seems to work for me.

During this talk, Tommy and memories of Tommy kept intruding as I went through my hour. Despite this, I stuck to my points and was told by various attendees that they enjoyed my remarks, so I guess I did the job I was supposed to do.

I left, went home, and didn't feel like doing much of anything for a couple of hours. Then I took myself out to dinner and had a large Manhattan with my meal. That seems to have helped.

I have lived in the same city with many of the same routines for decades. I am frequently in spaces that hold memories of Steve or Tommy. They're usually passing thoughts. This time was unusual, likely due to the nature of the association and the fact that I am rarely there.

Speaking of speaking, I have a bit of trepidation about the signing events and other book promotion stuff I have coming up. I'm fearless on stage when I'm in a role; directors can ask me to do pretty much anything. As long as I can make sense of the character and theatrical moments, I'll do it.

I've cursed, made racially insensitive jokes, appeared in nothing but body paint and a bunch of grapes, and other such things, and haven't thought much of it. But when it comes to just being me without a character to hide behind (and I count Dr. Duxbury as a character), I don't know what to do with myself.

I guess I'll have to develop an author persona I can conjure up for these things—an erudite, but warm individual who can act as psychic armor for those times when I'm not sure what's next.

I've always been terrible at self-promotion. There's something deep in my core that feels that no matter what I've achieved, it's not really worthy of any sort of attention. I suppose we all feel that way somewhat, at least in medicine.

One of the things I've always done with medical students is validated those sorts of feelings when they have them and explained that we all have them and that when they think their classmates have it all together and they do not, their classmates are thinking the exact same things about them.

The Delta wave continues to recede locally.

UAB's inpatient load is down to about half of what it was in late August, and there's nothing in the local numbers to suggest that it's about to accelerate again.

The Mountain West, however, remains exceedingly stressed.

They're a month or so behind where the Deep South was. Their October was our August. And still, so my sources tell me, the stubborn strain of COVID and vaccine denialism continues in those communities. There's going to be some serious long-term damage from this.

Hospitals and health systems, already stressed pre-pandemic by the fiscal realities of rural medicine, are going to start collapsing, leaving many communities without good local healthcare resources.

The psychic burdens, borne by the healthcare workers in these communities over the last couple of years as they have labored to care for their friends and neighbors, only to be reviled and scorned for accepting science over wishful thinking, cannot be borne long-term by anyone, and the human capital on which these institutions depend is going to melt away.

The older generation will retire. The younger generation will depart for greener pastures and communities where their skills and compassion are embraced and not spat upon.

⊱⊰

The big news of the last few days is twofold.

The first is that the FDA is well on its way to approving booster doses of both the Moderna and Johnson & Johnson formulations of COVID vaccines. I would expect both of them to be out and available by the end of the month.

Should you receive a booster?

The answer is yes if you fall into one of three major groups: (1) You have a disease process or take a medication that negatively impacts your immune system; (2) You have a job or other life pattern that brings you frequently into close contact with individuals of uncertain vaccination status; or (3) You are over the age of 65. Outside of those three groups, the answers are less clear. Talk to your physician.

I took mine as I fit into those categories. It didn't bother me any more than the original shots did. I also got my (regular) flu shot this week. It's a condition of my remaining gainfully employed.

The second bit of big news is that data has been submitted showing safety and efficacy of vaccination against COVID down to age five. Shots for children are also expected to be approved by the FDA shortly. This will allow all school-age children to be vaccinated and reduce some of the risks inherent in the school environment.

One would think that, as a society, we would make the health and well-being of our young of paramount importance. We did it with Polio and Smallpox vaccinations in the past, but we seem to be having more difficulty this time around.

The reasons for this have long and deep roots. I may consider a full essay on these later but the Manhattan tap-dancing through my central nervous system precludes my ability to do that tonight.

If I had children, I would be fighting like mad to get them vaccinated, but that doesn't seem to be a universal position. Some school districts and some states seem enamored of policies designed to appeal more to their parents' sense of righteous autonomy than to the safety and well-being of their charges.

I read the daily updates out of Florida and Texas, in particular, and all I can do now, after months of lunacy, is roll my eyes and move on. I suppose we're seeing the chattel origins of family life (where women and children were essentially the property of a man) continuing to play out through our social DNA.

If children are the property of their parents, then their parent's wishes are paramount and sacrosanct. If they wish them to be exposed to potentially fatal diseases, that is their right.

But we've moved away from that thinking over the last century or so to a view that children are also a societal good due to their potential to become functional and contributing adults. This has led us to invest in public education, child labor laws, child protective services, the frowning upon of corporal punishment, and the like.

Where the lines between a parent's wishes and society's needs should be drawn is ever-evolving and often somewhat murky. Children are removed every day from parents who use drugs, parents who are physically violent, parents of extreme religious beliefs who deny

382

their children medical care, and the like.

Is sending children to school without masks different? Is refusing vaccinations a form of child abuse? I don't have the answers to these questions, and the COVID pandemic, having happened and changing so quickly, hasn't really given us time to calm down, engage the issues rationally, and come together on common ground.

Too much thinking is making my head hurt!

Time to knock it off for the night. I wore my mask to my talk and only took it off on stage. I washed my hands. I kept my distance. I'm a good boy.

Most of the time.

MONDAY | OCTOBER 18, 2021

I HAVEN'T RUN THE NUMBERS FOR A WHILE.

We are definitely on the downside of the Delta wave locally with cases having fallen by nearly 50% in the last two weeks and fewer than 1,000 new diagnoses daily. Hospitalizations and deaths are also down with about 50 people dying a day in the state. That doesn't seem like much until you consider that's the equivalent of a jumbo jet crashing every week, and we are a relatively small state with only about five million people.

In 1982, seven people were murdered in the Chicago area with tampered Tylenol capsules. In the aftermath, we completely changed how goods are packaged, transported, and sold to prevent something similar from happening in the future. We're now at 726,000 US deaths from COVID and the response from a significant portion of the population is one of blasé nonchalance.

Indifference I get.

No matter how horrible the circumstances, life must be lived, work must be done, meals prepared, children tended to, like all the thousand-and-one other little details of our ordinary lives. Sometimes it's necessary to shut out the evils of the world in order to continue living.

What I don't get is those who are rising up in direct action and opposition to basic public health measures and good science, placing themselves and their families in harm's way. This is one I've been wrestling with for some time, trying to see if it fits into some logical narrative with other social trends.

"What about the children?" has become a cliché rallying cry, usually applied to some sort of ridiculous overreaction to a vaguely sensible social policy—oftentimes used to cover subjects to which children and child-rearing are only tangentially related at best.

This fetishization of childhood is a relatively new development in American culture. Earlier in American life, children were not regarded as innocents in need of protection from life but as neophytes who needed to be schooled in life's harsher realities so they could cope with tough times as an adult.

In agrarian America, children were a necessity to make sure enough produce could be wrested from the land to sustain the family through the winter. The children of the immigrant waves of the late 19th and early 20th centuries were put to work in dirty and dangerous occupations for pittances to help lift these new American families out of dire poverty and to ensure the profits of the owners of industry. Children's stories often included gruesome details and illustrations to help toughen them up.

The reforms of the Progressive Era of the early 20th century got kids out of factories and coal mines and into schools. The wrenching social changes of the World War I era helped spread new ideas of equality and the notion that education should go beyond the basics of literacy. The Depression and FDR's social reforms helped bring the country together in national identity over regional identity with an understanding that what was good for all was good for the individual.

The post-World War II prosperity spawned the Baby Boom, a generation that, in general, wanted for nothing and who were raised by parents traumatized by the horrific events of their formative years. Stories were Disneyfied, the new medium of television was sanitized, and history was whitewashed to protect this new generation of children from harsh realities.

As the Boom matured, they rebelled, leading to the massive cultural changes of the 60s and 70s. But they have always carried with them a nostalgia for a more perfect time—one that never actually existed outside the tropes of mass media—and have passed this on to their children and grandchildren.

I think some of the current actions and reactions regarding the protection of children from the very real dangers of COVID are caught up in all of this. Anti-vaccination movements, while present, never really caught on when the standard vaccines for such diseases as polio, measles, and whooping cough appeared in the 50s and 60s. Parents of the era, having known bad times, were more than eager to protect their children by any means necessary, and childhood vaccines passed into the common wisdom without much fuss.

When the Boomers and Gen X grew up and became parents themselves, things changed. Some of this was due to the ideas of alternative healing that took off in the 70s. Some of this was due to the rise of mass media platforms. Some of this was due to celebrity culture in which well-known individuals used their influence to peddle ideas with no basis in fact but which gained traction anyway.

The modern anti-vaccination movement started to gain steam in the early 1980s when a reporter named Lea Thompson (not the actress) produced a documentary called DPT: Vaccine Roulette which linked the vaccine, using flimsy and circumstantial evidence, to a host of health problems in children.

Lawsuits against vaccine manufacturers by parents of disabled children began to skyrocket, and manufacturers warned Congress that if they weren't protected, they would get out of the business. Congress, concerned that vaccines might become unaffordable or unavailable, passed the National Childhood Vaccine Injury Act in 1986 which more or less shielded vaccine manufacturers from liability regarding their products.

In 1990, the Vaccine Adverse Event Reporting System (VAERS) was created to take reports and track issues with vaccines. While there is a lot of data in VAERS, it is voluntarily self-reported and not systematized, making it very difficult to draw conclusions or under-stand trends in a sound epidemiologic manner.

Also during this period, Dr. Robert Mendelsohn, one of the first anti-vaccine pediatricians, wrote a book decrying vaccination which was taken seriously in some circles. Dr. Mendelsohn also decried the evils of fluoridation, coronary artery bypass grafting, and breast can-cer screening, so I don't take him very seriously myself.

The rise of the daytime talk format in the late 80s and early 90s, pioneered by Phil Donahue and then taken into new areas of social argument by Morton Downey Jr., gave a forum to such noted scientists and health educators as Jenny McCarthy and Lisa Bonet who appeared multiple times decrying vaccines as unnatural micro-organisms responsible for sudden infant death, brain damage, autism, and other ills, despite having no evidence for any of these claims. Well-to-do par-ents on the left latched on to the unnatural idea, and vaccine rates be-gan to decline in wealthy liberal neighborhoods throughout the 1990s.

Another turning point came in 1998 when British physician An-drew Wakefield published an article in the medical journal *The Lancet*, linking the MMR vaccine with the development of autism. This particular paper captured public attention and entered the zeitgeist where it remains, despite the fact that the study was falsified, the journal retracted the paper, and Dr. Wakefield lost his medical license.

Over the last generation, the advent of social media has allowed for the amplification of alternative voices and has allowed anti-vaccine communities to come together, share resources, and recruit others to their belief system.

A major driver has been society's anger at Big Pharma and the outrageous price gouging that has become a standard part of their business model over the last few decades. Vaccines have become an easy target for people frustrated over their inability to afford health care or cope with an increasingly complex and unfriendly health system.

When it is obvious that a public good such as health care is not operating in the public interest, it becomes easy to ascribe nefarious motives as to why this is. Conspiracy theory thinking takes hold. Eventually, some begin to believe that the manufacturers of vaccines are incapable of telling the truth or acting in the public interest.

Where is all this going?

I think if we see where anti-vaccination sentiment comes from, it becomes easier to understand the mindset of those who hold it. They see themselves as holding the line against a corrupt system that does not actually have the health of America as its chief interest, and I can't say that they are completely wrong in that idea.

What is a bit harder for me is how this translates into anti-mask and anti-distancing sentiment. Those ideas are common sense that have been proven time and again to control the spread of pandemic disease going back millennia.

Perhaps our education system, after 20 years of No Child Left Behind and teaching only to standardized tests, has created a generation incapable of critical thought and incurious enough to look up even basic historical information, despite a portal in their pocket to much of human knowledge. Perhaps the politics of anti-vaccination, in an attempt to draw tribal lines against pro-vaccinators, blurred the boundaries between various public health precautions making all of them suspect.

The educated classes directing the *lumpenproletariat* have all been vaccinated of course. It's a rather cynical move of theirs not to correct the thinking of their followers but rather abandon them to the realities of infectious disease. Rupert Murdoch, for instance, took a private jet to Great Britain to get a vaccination the first week they became available. He's 90 years old and not a fool.

While it would be easy to demonize those arguing against public health measures as Phoenicians offering up their children as sacrifices to Kronos, it's not that simple. Nothing ever is. All I can do is wonder, try to be on the right side of the argument based on what I know of medicine and health, and keep my hands washed and my mask on indoors.

SUNDAY | OCTOBER 24, 2021

T'S BEEN SIX DAYS SINCE I WROTE A LONG PIECE.

In my head, it's coming out in Gloria Stuart's Old Rose voice along the lines of "It's been 85 years…" as if there's something seriously wrong if I don't churn out some piece of gentle wisdom a couple of times a week.

Nothing's wrong.

All is as well as can be expected within the borders of Andydom.

I just went to the theater and the movies this weekend rather than staying home and writing a think piece.

><0>

Local numbers continue to decline.

The number of hospitalized patients at UAB this weekend is down to a couple of dozen, about the same as it was early in the summer before the numbers began to skyrocket with Delta variant infections.

I am under no illusions that we're done with COVID, though.

Vaccination rates remain significantly below where they should be and, with that remaining the case, we're still sitting ducks for the next variant that improves transmissibility or causes more serious illness than those that are currently circulating.

I don't know if the health system can survive another wave or two.

The majority of practitioners of my generation are making their exit plans, burned out by the experiences of the last 18 months; the younger ones, who still have time to revamp their careers, are starting to look at less stressful ways of making a living.

I don't think we're going to run out of doctors in the near future, and medical school class slots are hardly going begging; it's the positions that allow doctors to actually do their jobs that are becoming harder and harder to fill: nursing, medical assistants, nurse's aides, and all the other support staff.

Finding quality candidates for good jobs at both UAB and the VA is starting to become more and more difficult. I've had conversations with healthcare entities outside of my big systems, and they're having an even tougher time finding the staff they need.

This is going to create a major issue in the next decade as aging Baby Boomers, whether they believe it or not, ate going to start having to deal with the chronic illnesses and infirmities of age, and are going to start requiring professional assistance to maintain their lives.

The big four issues of aging are meals, wheels, bills, and pills.

This is what I teach my residents to check into when they have an older patient. They're part of what we call the instrumental activities of daily living in the biz. These are in contrast to the basic activities of daily living; the things you have to be able to do to maintain your own body. Most of us have been pretty good with these since about age five. Anyone who gets out of bed in the morning, heads into the bathroom, and gets ready for the day on their own has got them covered.

Twenty years ago, there were roughly 30 million Americans over 65. Of these, about five million required assistance from someone to maintain their lives in the community. Another one-and-a-half million lived in a nursing facility.

These days, we're at about 50 million Americans over 65. They've actually become more functional. Nursing home residents are down to about 1.3 million. 'A smaller percentage depends on help at home. However, the rise in population has drowned out these gains. We're up to about seven-and-a-half million people needing help at home.

In 2030, eight years from now, these numbers will go up substantially as the older Boomers start to enter their late 80s and the great Boomer die-off of 2030-2050 begins. And they're likely to need more in-home workers due to cultural shifts of the last half-century.

More Boomers are entering elderhood single than in previous generations. Something like 60% of women over 80 live alone.

Children are fewer and more apt to live in a different geographical area than their parents. Informal networks like clubs and churches are less strong as people have withdrawn into suburban cocoons.

This means the demand for paid help in the home is going to grow exponentially just at a time when the industry is shedding workers due to the changes wrought by COVID.

These are the kinds of side effects that those who are blithely ignoring public health measures, or who have chosen political stances incompatible with good social order, are not considering when they make their defiant proclamations. Their decisions, which allow for a deadly virus to keep circulating and stressing the healthcare system, will keep the healthcare system from functioning as it should.

≈

The system has had serious issues for decades due to its business models. If the people who keep it propped up abandon it for easier careers or retirement or just because of plain old burnout, what then?

If the number of skilled providers of in-home support and health services declines as the population ages, Adam Smith's laws of supply and demand suggest that these services will only be available to the wealthiest. If nursing homes cannot hire staff and are cited by governmental regulators, corporate owners will close them as bad investments and no one will want to open new ones.

Governmental entities could potentially close the gap, but there's no interest these days in raising taxes to enhance social services. The current infrastructure bill is, in general, funded in ways other than tax increases. But this sleight of hand can't be kept up forever.

If we returned to the tax schedule of the pre-Reagan 1970s, we would have collected $26 trillion over the last 40 years for the common good. Instead, it went into private hands. Staying out of disastrous military adventures would have garnered us another 15 trillion or so. We the people decided to go a different way, so we the people must live with the consequences of those decisions.

Most of us don't have the resources we will need for old age. Current estimates are that the Baby Boom generation will need between three and four hundred thousand dollars apiece for healthcare expenses not covered by Medicare.

We can usually thrive if our bodies and brains will allow us to remain independent. For those of us where this is no longer possible, the costs of long-term care are astronomical and not covered by Medicare. They are covered by Medicaid if you are impoverished, at least on paper, but as these costs rise rapidly in state budgets, states are actively looking at ways to shift them back onto the population at large.

If you want someone to come into your home and assist, figure $15-25 an hour for non-skilled care. If it's a skilled nurse, double that. If you want to live in a senior community with assistance, figure $3,500-5,500 a month plus buy-in fees for the more upscale. If you need to live in a nursing home, figure $5,000-7,000 a month.

The average liquid asset life savings for an American retiring today is just over $100,000. That'll buy you about 15 months of nursing home care. The average person who enters a nursing home for long-term care is there for between four and five years.

There is much I could say about nursing home care. There are many wonderful people dedicated to the field who do the best they can. The way the industry runs, however, is not friendly to innovation or the support of good employees. But that's a subject for a different rant on a different day.

I didn't have any idea when I began this piece that it was going to be about long-term care. It's just what came out this evening.

All I can hope is that those, especially those in significant positions of power, who continue to defy public health and logic, are going to be prepared to deal with the mess when the other dominos start to fall.

The attorney general of Alabama has been grandstanding again that Alabama won't let employers, or those offering services to the public, mandate vaccination. He and the governor can posture all they want but UAB, the largest employer in the state, is mandating vaccination. They have to. It's a requirement for all federal contractors via executive order, and UAB isn't about to leave tens of millions of dollars on the table so some yahoos in Montgomery can bloviate in front of television cameras.

My other major employer, the VA, is also mandating vaccination as the same executive order is requiring it of all federal employees. I'm glad I can go to work and not have to worry too much about who I'm passing in the halls.

Meanwhile, Governor DeSantis is trying to get a $5,000 bonus payment to hire out-of-state police officers who refuse vaccination and have them come to work in Florida. I'm not sure that filling the police departments of Florida full of vaccine deniers is the wisest of ideas, especially in this time of increased public scrutiny of bad behavior by the police—but that's just me.

I have a feeling that the state of Florida will end up paying some very large settlements after a certain type of bad apple moves in and goes to work. The voters of Florida are getting what they voted for. It'll be interesting to see if they keep voting that way in the future.

I could keep on with this drivel for a few more paragraphs, but I'm due at a birthday celebration, so I'm going to sign off. Yes, I'll wear my mask and wash my hands. And I've had my booster.

SATURDAY | OCTOBER 30, 2021

I T'S BEEN A LUGUBRIOUS COUPLE OF DAYS: dreary and gray with intermittent rain showers. Very Seattle.

Such weather used to make me homesick, but as I haven't lived in Seattle for nearly 35 years, that phase has passed. Now it merely makes me sleepy.

I came home from work yesterday, sat down on the bed with every intention of doing some writing, and woke up four hours later. Of course, this meant that when it was actually time to go to bed, I was bouncing off the walls. I ended up staying awake most of the night, binge-watching old episodes of *Supernatural*.

I'll get myself back on track over the weekend. I don't have much scheduled other than a Halloween party tonight. I have a feeling I will make an appearance but not stay too late.

We haven't run the numbers for a bit.

We're at just over 745,000 deaths in the US and just about to hit five million deaths worldwide. The world figure is a major undercount as there are significant parts of the globe without access to appropriate testing to know whether deaths are related to coronavirus or not.

The Delta Wave is pretty much on the downslide both locally and nationally, but we're not out of the woods. Nationally, we're still losing somewhere between 1000 and 1500 people a day which is a good deal higher than the numbers of this past spring when the rollout of vaccine and better social behavior were driving spread way down.

And then there was Delta.

I'm waiting for another strain to start spreading as we still have a large unvaccinated reservoir in the US population. In Alabama, we're up to about 2/3 of adults having at least one vaccine and 55% being fully vaccinated. It's better than it was, but there's still a long way to go.

The senior population is doing much better. In Alabama, nearly 90% of those over 65 have had at least one shot, and more than three-quarters are fully vaccinated. I can breathe a little easier about my patient population.

Nationwide, 97% of those over 65 have had at least one shot and nearly 90% are fully vaccinated. Despite being heavy consumers of Fox News and other propaganda outlets, they understood the risks to them and their health.

The prevalence of vaccination in this age group means that the Delta wave did not really do much damage to older Americans. The death rate over the last six months for them is comparable to other respiratory viral illnesses such as influenza or respiratory syncytial virus.

Delta killed, and is still killing, the middle-aged who decided to put politics and tribal identity ahead of their own health concerns. Older adults have memories of prior pandemic diseases such as polio and the miracle wrought by the public health vaccination campaigns of the 40s through the 70s.

Those under 60 may recall getting their shots but would have no real adult memory of the rise and fall of epidemic disease. Never having experienced it, to them it's not quite real. It's a relic of a bygone time like the grainy black and white photographs of the two World Wars. So when pandemic disease showed its ugly head in the modern era, younger generations were not prepared to process what was happening to them and their society.

In that liminal space between events and reactions, various forces took root, urged on by a political system that thrives on controversy, one-upmanship, and a sort of high stakes football game with each side trying to move the ball to their own end of the field and tackling the opposing side as they do so.

And here we are.

I don't foresee us really being out of the pandemic until next spring, although many of my living patterns, as they happen in a segment of society with very high levels of vaccination, are returning to what they were pre-COVID.

Viruses are sneaky and, as they are such simple organisms, they are constantly mutating. Sometimes those mutations are fortuitous for the virus to begin spreading anew or to create more serious illness in the host. I have a feeling we've got another wave or two to come. As vaccination levels are going up, albeit slowly, new waves may not be as serious as the Delta wave of this summer.

As I presumed, the government has not mandated vaccines on the population. They have, however, mandated them on federal employees and contractors as a condition of employment. The government doesn't want sick employees and quarantines to interrupt its business any more than it has to. It doesn't want sick or quarantined military troops.

The troops that are fussing about the vaccine are being a little silly. They had to have all sorts of vaccines as part of their induction into service, including things like anthrax to protect against biological warfare agents. Now they're complaining?

State and local governments in blue areas are also mandating that public employees, especially first responders, health workers, and school employees be vaccinated. In most areas, there is grumbling, but when people realize their job is on the line, they get vaccinated and they are fine. The hospitals of Los Angeles are not overrun with school district employees suffering serious vaccine complications.

In red states, they are busy passing laws preventing local govern-ments from mandating vaccines for public employees and are searching for ways to nullify the federal mandates.

They won't have much luck.

There is well over a century of precedent allowing such actions in public health emergencies, and the few COVID-related questions that have reached our conservative Supreme Court have been turned away in favor of vaccination.

The private world, with our ridiculous employment-based health insurance system, has realized that they will be on the hook for many expensive hospitalizations if vaccination is not widespread. Big companies are coming down firmly on the side of vaccination as a condition of employment.

No, it's not a violation of your rights for them to do this. They can mandate all sorts of things regarding your job such as uniforms, dress code, safety policies, etc. This is just one more thing in that long list.

If you cannot abide by your employer's rules, you are free to seek employment elsewhere or to become self-employed and set your own rules. Some large companies are not allowing sick leave to be used for COVID quarantine if you are unvaccinated, making it time off without pay.

I suspect that the insurance plans offered in 2022 when people go through their annual open enrollment a year from now, will have a new rider denying coverage for COVID claims in the unvaccinated who cannot prove medical contraindication or long-standing religious belief regarding vaccine use.

━━⊱◈⊰━━

Where will all this leave us?

I think it means that the next inevitable wave of COVID will be confined to rural and suburban areas in states which have not taken vaccination seriously for political reasons.

Most city dwellers, whether in red or blue states, are vaccinated, so even though population density is higher in cities, the virus will have less purchase, especially if we keep up the new patterns we have developed of moving, dining, and other social activities outside as much as the weather permits.

As more and more data becomes available, it's becoming increasingly clear that the virus is not easily transmitted in outdoor environments (or indoor environments with high airflow). It's also not particularly well transmitted on surfaces. So you can let the kids trick or treat outside and you don't have to Clorox the candy. The new normal should be for the adults to sit on the porch with the candy bowl to hand it out rather than forcing kids to come all the way to the front door.

<hr>

The weather is changing. (This is where we came in on this essay.) And with that, social behavior is going to start changing, too; we're going to move more indoors. Then we have the holidays with the usual gatherings and travel patterns.

Will this lead to a fresh wave this winter? I'm hoping there's enough vaccine out there that we'll see a little blip up but not a steep curve as we had in July and August with Delta.

Time will tell.

If Halloween parties make an impact, we'll be seeing rates of hospitalization increase again in mid-November. The effects of Thanksgiving will become apparent in mid-December. Christmas cheer and New Year's celebrations will make themselves known by mid-to-late January.

Assuming I haven't gone completely barmy, I'll report back on all this when the time comes.

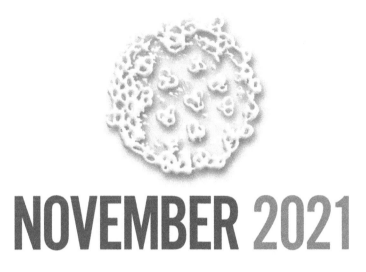

NOVEMBER 2021

From This Moment On

THURSDAY | NOVEMBER 4, 2021

WENT TO SEE A PRODUCTION OF *The Glass Menagerie* this evening in the small black box space at the theater where I have done most of my work in musicals—19 shows over the 17 years since I made my debut there in *Jekyll and Hyde* as the butler.

For years, the word was out: need a butler, a random aristocrat, a drunk? Call Andy.

I'm generally not a huge Tennessee Williams fan but the scaling down of the piece to fit the intimate space made me really listen to the language and how beautiful the choice of words is. I'm a reasonable writer but then I see something like that and I realize how inadequate my little scribblings are.

I was dwelling on the famous closing speech Tom gives in which he says nowadays the world is lit by lightning. Blow out your candles, Laura. And so, goodbye. I was coming up the hill back to my condo and thought perhaps there's something terribly prescient in that sentiment.

We are living through a time of great change, a time that is indeed lit by lightning, and those who attempt to sit back amid the candles of the past are doomed to a slow fade into oblivion.

The lightning strikes and peals of thunder are, to a certain extent, created by the monster of the 24-hour news cycle that's come to dominate political and social discourse over the last few decades. In the past, you got your news in the form of the daily paper. It was formatted in such a way that you could take it in slowly and digest it with your breakfast or your before-dinner cocktail. If it was a bit assaultive, you could always turn to the comics, the sports section, or the arts and entertainment pages.

The only available visual news was pretty much limited to half-hour local and half-hour national newscasts that stuck to facts rather than opinion due to the strictures of the Fairness Doctrine. Things have changed a bit with the invention of continuous cable news networks, the demise of the daily paper, and the availability of insta-news of dubious quality via various online sources distributed through social media.

There's something in the American character that loves competition. Not just competition, brutal winner-take-all competition.

It's no wonder that football took off here and not in any other country. The idea of a sort of gladiatorial combat in which men maul at each other to capture territory, and which is set up so that only one team can be the champion and get the accolades, seems to fit in with the country built on manifest destiny and the rolling over and exploiting of the less fortunate and less powerful.

I've never been a big football fan. This has not served me particularly well since moving to Alabama where football is a religion.

I joke about the sportsball, but I do usually know who's winning and losing. You can't avoid it in this part of the country.

I attended football games in the student section when I was in college. I brought a book. My college career did give me my one and only football claim to fame. I was there in the stands in 1982 for the Stanford v. Cal game that included the crazy finale with the infamous "band play." I saw the trombonist get tackled. It was wild.

We all know that the most interesting sports competitions are those which are the closest. It's the suspense of not having a foregone conclusion—the last-minute field goal, the impossible save—that grabs and keeps our attention and gives us something to talk about for the next week until there's a new highlight.

These sort of edge-of-the-seat moments are great in the sporting world, but in this brave new world of fleeting attention spans, these qualities are invading other areas of our lives. In an attempt to capture our eyeballs, however briefly, mass media is causing certain areas of our lives to become counterproductive.

Take the movies, for instance.

Reportage on film used to be about the quality of the product, written by critics of discernment. Now it's all about who captured the box office and is number one or how many teenagers paid to see the latest MCU opus opening weekend.

The language is full of sporting and military metaphors. The result has been a significant decline of lower-budget films *about* adults *for* adults as they can't possibly "beat" the competition and "win" the weekend.

This has become most corrosive in our politics, especially on a national level.

Politics and governance are not inherently exciting subjects. In the past, no one was terribly interested in what went on behind the closed doors of Congressional meeting rooms as the sausage was being made. People were much more interested in what was presented after the wheeling and dealing was over and policy was voted upon.

Congress was there to do the people's business and to get policies with popular support enacted into legislation. Now, most Congresspeople seem to be acting out of a sense of personal aggrandizement. As the old adage goes, politics is show business for the unattractive.

The media, needing to create the news cycle and excitement to get the clicks and the eyeballs, spins as much as possible into a continuous horse race between red and blue where they're constantly neck and neck, calling first for one side, then the other. The result is a dishonest look at the business of governing— a continued push to pick a team and team colors, and to be yelling for your team from your side of the stands.

This has spread even to what should be apolitical topics such as public health.

There have always been people opposed to public health measures, but they have generally not been given a megaphone to spread their ideas, and their ideas have generally gone dormant once the public at large has seen the benefits of vaccination/sanitation/industrial safety/smoking reduction or whatever other issue is at the forefront.

With the recent introduction of coronavirus vaccines, the sentiment seems to be everywhere. If you go back through the various streams of information, most of the anti-vaccine rhetoric comes from a surprisingly few outlets—fewer than 20 in total.

The most incendiary and outrageous ideas get magnified by social media and then the news media as a whole picks up on them. Then the nature of the news cycle and the need for the close horse race takes over. Before we know it, a small minority opinion based on spurious assertion seems to have equal weight with a large majority opinion that has all the facts and science on its side.

This is, I suppose, why the media predicted that tens of thousands of NYPD officers would leave their jobs rather than take the vaccine when required. The actual number who have left so far is fewer than 50.

Tying vaccine status to job/salary, whether you agree with it or not, is working to bring the numbers of vaccinated up relatively rapidly and, concomitantly, hospitalization rates are going down. At UAB today, we're down to ten COVID inpatients. To my knowledge, there aren't any hospitalizations there due to vaccine side effects.

I don't know what to do about any of this any more than anyone else does.

All I can do is recognize the patterns and hopefully continue to read widely and deeply on current affairs from multiple perspectives, avoid television news and clickbait, and not put too much stock into the results of any particular partisan race having a whole lot of meaning for the future of the country as a whole.

I've also had my shots and my booster. I've kept my hands washed. And I wore my mask in the theater.

MONDAY | NOVEMBER 8, 2021

THE WEEKEND WAS BUSY and the workweek promises to be busier still.

I thought the change in time might fix my chronic fatigue, but alas, this has not come to pass. I'm still feeling very drawn out.

I have a new understanding of Bilbo Baggins' line about feeling spread too thin like not enough butter on the toast in *The Fellowship of the Ring*. I better check my jewelry to see if anything has a previously unknown power.

I don't wear a lot of jewelry. Cuff links with dressing up, the occasional ring. I took my wedding ring off a few months after Tommy died and put it away in the box where I keep my other pieces. I look at it occasionally and remember, but I don't want to look at it all day every day as I have in the past. Gotta keep moving on.

The night after seeing *The Glass Menagerie*, I went out to Encore Theater, the African-American theater company run by a friend, to see a production of Dominique Morisseau's *Skeleton Crew* (shortly coming to Broadway in a production starring Phylicia Rashad).

Like *The Glass Menagerie*, it's an intimate four-person drama served best by a small house connecting audience and actors. But the two plays could not be more different stylistically or in subject matter.

Skeleton Crew is an unflinching look at four African-American Detroit autoworkers at a manufacturing plant threatened by the economic downturn of 2008. I enjoyed it very much and thought that all four of the performers were exceptional in their roles.

I hope more of the theater community will check out the Encore and its productions. Everything I've seen there has been top-notch in terms of the performances, and I've learned a great deal by turning up there regularly. If they ever need an old white guy for something they're mounting, they'll know who to ask.

It continued to be a theatrical weekend with my having to get up early Saturday morning and head out into the hinterlands to be a judge for the Alabama high school theater competition, known as Trumbauer, after a Walter Trumbauer who I assume did something at some point to get the whole thing off the ground.

This year, my category was musical theater duets—both dramatic and comedic. Some very good, some not so. They're mainly 14 to 17-year-old kids, so one always gives them an "A" for effort and looks for constructive ways to help them improve.

I've done this every year I can for a decade or so. I always enjoy it. I've seen some of the more skilled participants eventually join the cadre of performers in the greater Birmingham area, sharing their talents beyond school audiences.

We have a talented theater community here. We have folk with extensive professional credits who have ended up in Birmingham for family or other personal reasons but still want to perform. We have theater kids who have gone on to major careers in New York and elsewhere. Local folk I've worked with are currently playing the title role in *Dear Evan Hansen* and Simba in *The Lion King*. Another is understudying Sutton Foster in the new production of *The Music Man*.

My next major theatrical moment of the weekend was trooping down to the Virginia Samford Theater for a callback for Larry in

Sondheim's *Company*. I don't expect to get it for various reasons but being considered competitive for a role in a Sondheim show is a huge ego boost.

One of my friends in New York was a member of the original Broadway cast of *Company* as one of the vocal minority, so I asked her to send me some long-distance good mojo. I also shared that the sentence "I have been called back for the role of Larry in *Company*" is not one I would ever expect to write.

I am acutely aware of my limitations as a musician, singer, and performer, in general. If I am cast, I will work like hell to rise to the demands of the piece, the character, and the production, but it's very hard work preparing for roles where I feel like I'm outside my comfort zone. It's good for me to stretch, however, and maybe bite off a bit more than I can chew.

Lastly, I spent 90 minutes on stage as myself doing a reading from Volume One of *The Accidental Plague Diaries* and an interview regarding its creation as a benefit for Central Alabama Theater.

I generally don't get stage fright. As long as I feel like I'm adequately rehearsed and prepared, I just go out there and do my thing. That was not true this time. I was very nervous about getting up there with no character and no one else's words to hide behind. I'm told the whole thing went well but to me, it was a bit of a blur.

COVID is receding locally into the background. I am under no illusions that it's going to stay there. This virus is hardy and sneaky, and it rapidly mutates, so there's still more to come. With international travel picking back up, variants will have lots of opportunities to jump borders and into new populations with relative ease. I wish I could predict what's coming next, but I can't.

Many things are happening, any of which could significantly affect the next stage of the pandemic. These include the vaccination of children. Children 11-and-under are one of the last great pools of unvaccinated individuals and, as the vaccine rolls out to them over the next few weeks, that may change how transmission chains work.

We're just about to enter the holiday season with the annual travel and gatherings of family and friends. With last year having been a bust, there may be redoubled efforts to get people together this year, especially in families that have been vaccinated. They're unlikely to make each other sick, but there's always that chance of spreading subclinical disease which may then be carried to an unvaccinated population elsewhere.

The weather is changing, driving people indoors. Much social activity was redirected outside over the spring and summer as people recognized it was much safer, but that trend may not last with colder weather. Case numbers are going up again in Northern Europe. The change in weather is thought to be one of the reasons why.

Then there's corporate America and policies tying vaccine status to employability. Trends so far suggest that only a small minority are willing to put their livelihood on the line to avoid the vaccine.

Data continues to pour in on safety and efficacy. The major risk factor currently in the US for being unvaccinated is political party affiliation. A recent analysis shows that those in predominantly red counties are three times as likely to die as those in predominantly blue counties. When you drill down on the data, that differential is almost all due to vaccine hesitancy among Republicans.

The US death toll topped 750,000 this week.

It was roughly 375,000 on New Year's Day, so the 2021 death toll is now the same as it was in 2020, and we still have two months to go. This shouldn't have happened as we've had a safe and effective vaccine for all of 2021. It wasn't widely available early in the year, but as of April or May it's been pretty much everywhere.

The social rules of belonging to one of two competing Americas, red or blue, have prevented the effective use of vaccines. Today, a sitting US senator attacked Big Bird from Sesame Street for spreading propaganda for some mild statements regarding vaccination.

Big Bird has been a tool of American public health in explaining and demystifying vaccines for children since 1972 and has flown under the radar (so to speak) for nearly 50 years. Why the faux outrage now? Especially from a senator who has himself been vaccinated.

Historians of the future, trying to parse the current times in a century or two, are going to be very puzzled about all of this. The portion of the population that rejects education, expertise, science, health, and other sundry items in an attempt to define itself by being the antithesis of the other side is going to have a very difficult time creating policies allowing the US to function in the modern world the next time they come to power.

And they will come to power again—it's the way the US political system works. Its winner-take-all structure pretty much foreordains a two-party system with power see-sawing between them at fairly regular intervals. If we want something different, we're going to have to elect a different sort of Congress. I don't think the monied interests who pay for campaigns are going to be very interested in that.

><>

This week, outside of the usual work stuff, I have two depositions to prepare for my medicolegal side gig. I'd rather not be doing this, but deadlines and court dates approach.

This work provides a little more money I can donate to help get the local arts community back on its feet following pandemic catastrophes. But I might just keep a little for myself this time for a new trip.

Signing off for the night. You all know the drill. Wash your hands, wear your mask indoors unless everyone's vaccinated, don't go out if you're sick with anything, and support your local arts community.

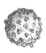

FRIDAY | NOVEMBER 12, 2021

HAVE THE FEELING that I better write this evening.

I'm not sure what this is going to be about but there's something stirring deep in my limbic system, banging on the thalamus, demanding to get out. I haven't identified it yet. Perhaps it will make itself known as I sit here and type.

I don't think it's about work as the week was relatively quiet. My clinic patients were predominantly well, the VA had a Thursday federal holiday so I had yesterday off—a rare occurrence for me (I slept in and played catch up on a number of projects around the condo), and the deposition I had been prepping for all week was canceled at the last minute.

If all my work weeks were like this, I could easily continue working into my 80s but this is the exception and not the rule. When my patients notice my aging, they look at me with an accusing glare, daring me to retire before they're done with me. I'm now nearly 25 years older than I was when I started at UAB, and I still care for some of the same people—in their 70s then, their 90s now.

The side effects of COVID on the healthcare system are driving a lot of my generation into earlier than originally planned retirement. In fact, some of the "great resignation" that's being talked about with workers not returning from the last year and a half of catastrophe is older workers deciding that it's just not worth it to go back to the stresses of jobs after a prolonged chance of figuring out other patterns of living.

This is particularly true of health care given the inherent dangers of the field during a pandemic plus the precarious nature of a previously rickety system having been subjected to mind-boggling stresses. It's sort of like a beach cabin that's been in the family for generations, much loved, but not necessarily kept up as well as it might have been—and then a Category 5 hurricane hits. It may still be standing after the storm, but it won't necessarily be as sturdy or as functional as it once was.

Most nurses, therapists, and other professionals over the age of 60 are mapping out their exit strategies, and there just aren't enough talented younger folk to replace them. I wonder sometimes if my clinical fiefdom at UAB could survive my retirement.

Both nationally and locally there is a dearth of physicians with any interest in geriatric medicine, and the economics of the system are such that it's nigh on impossible to make geriatric ambulatory care pay for itself. Not to mention that providing outpatient care in geriatrics is hard and the clinical schedules for outpatient work are rigid and punishing.

><>

Local COVID numbers continue to trend positively with fewer than 500 new diagnoses daily and few of those requiring hospitalization.

The national trends are not as rosy.

We're still losing between 1100 and 1200 people a day. This may not sound like much until you multiply it out and realize that it's more than 400,000 people a year—more than have died in either 2020 or, to date, in 2021.

The hot spots have shifted in the last few weeks away from the Deep South and the Mississippi River Valley to the Mountain West, the Great Lakes Region, and Northern New England. For instance, case rates in Vermont, one of the most vaccinated states, are skyrocketing. Its small size and population mean that the absolute numbers of sick or dead are quite small, but the percentages are concerning.

If I had to make a guess, I'm thinking we are seeing the results of the change in seasons. All of the places where numbers are going up are places where the temperature drops and winter sets in early. This forces people indoors, and I'm thinking that more people indoors around other people more often may be the driver. This would also explain why case rates have been increasing in Northern Europe but not in Southern Europe.

If this is true, we're going to see a big spike following gatherings for Thanksgiving—which will likely be very popular this year due to the inability to do so last year and general COVID fatigue among the population.

Fortunately, the vaccines seem to be doing their job. COVID breakthrough cases in the vaccinated are uncommon, though not rare, and the vast majority seem to cause mild illness requiring minimal treatment unless the individual has other significant health conditions. Unvaccinated adults remain at relatively high risk of serious illness, hospitalization, and death.

More and more data are coming out showing that the disease burden is concentrating itself in unvaccinated communities and that these can be mapped to political belief. The latest piece of nonsense to appear is some quack advocating COVID detoxification baths with Epsom salts, borax, and other such things to kill the nanobots. Someone watched the latest James Bond film a few too many times.

At least this one is relatively harmless, unlike injecting bleach, gargling with betadine, or eating horse deworming paste, but it does show a complete misunderstanding of what the vaccines are, how they work, and what they actually do in your system. I suppose it's so that those who get the vaccine as it becomes more and more tied to employment can get it and then immerse themselves in a ritual mikvah to wash away the uncleanliness of it all and return purified to their tribe.

I'm still working out the risks I'm personally willing to take.

I wear my mask indoors around other people unless we're all vaccinated or I'm actively eating and drinking. As this is a red state with minimal guidance from the top for political reasons, every venue and organization is more or less left to its own devices to try and determine best practices.

The opera is requiring masking at indoor events unless eating or drinking. One theater company in town is requiring proof of vaccination or a negative test to enter. Another suggests masks but doesn't enforce them, and I was one of the few audience members who remained masked the last time I attended a show.

Fortunately, the sort of people who make up live theater/classical music audiences are the sort of people who are likely to have been vaccinated, so I'm not overly worried.

These days, I'm regularly applying what I call the car test: Is what I do riskier than getting in an automobile on a routine basis?

The current chance of dying in an auto accident per year in the US is 12.4/100,000 population. The chance of a vaccinated individual dying of COVID is 0.1/100,000 population, so I'm not worried about keeling over.

At this point, I'm willing to return to theater life, but with a dollop of common sense. I'm keeping my hands washed. I'm keeping my mask on unless actively performing. I've had my shots and my booster and most theaters are insisting that their performers all provide proof of vaccination.

The first show I have booked is *The Eight: The Reindeer Monologues* as Comet. It's eight solo monologues, rehearsal contacts will be minimal, and I can stay six feet away from the audience.

Tommy and I went to see the show a number of years ago when Birmingham Festival Theater last did it.

I wonder what he'd think of me being in it? He was always quietly encouraging of my stage career, just as long as it never interfered with his schedule or things he wanted to do.

WEDNESDAY | NOVEMBER 17, 2021

'M A BIT ON EDGE TONIGHT.

The last day or so has been seesawing between minor wins and little losses. I don't know if it's pandemic coping exhaustion or something else. But little things have been pushing me toward lassitude.

I've spent the last few hours feeling like I could fall asleep on my feet even though it's not been a particularly arduous day. The way I put it together is as follows.

We've all been stewing in a toxic environment of danger signals for some years now.

Turn on the TV? Some pundit with excess jowls, too much foundation, and an inability to remain the least bit calm begins to deliver a highly opinionated tale of doom and gloom. Browse social media? Clickbait headlines announce imminent disasters of various kinds. Phone a friend? You'll eventually get around to some story of a mutual acquaintance who became seriously ill with COVID or with post-infection Long COVID symptoms.

A constant mental diet of this is revving up our limbic systems and primitive brain functions into a high state of alertness. Our brains, evolved for a hunter-gatherer savannah life, don't understand that the saber-tooth tiger isn't about to come over the hill, and are forcing us into a certain level of paralysis in order to conserve energy to fight or flee the physical danger they assume will arrive at any moment.

Must stay still. Must conserve energy resources. Must hold on to extra energy in case we have to walk great distances to greener pastures.

That's why we've all gained weight and are having difficulty shedding the extra pounds. To our primitive brains, that fat is energy storage for when the ever-promised danger arrives and we need extra strength and stamina to survive.

⤜

Mental health is deteriorating everywhere due to all of this, and I assume we're going to have enormous amounts of depression, anxiety disorders, and post-traumatic stress issues to deal with as a society for some years going forward. Add this to the physical toll of Long COVID which is likely to render a significant number of people unable to function as independent adults without assistance from others.

And where are the nurturers and the caregivers and the mental health professionals supposed to come from? These fields have always been poorly paid and low on the social totem pole due to their identification with a traditionally female workforce and feminine characteristics.

Job categories that require traditionally male attributes such as aggression, autonomy, and precision, and which have been generally reserved for males prior to the social changes of 50 to 60 years ago, have always been considered more important than those that require traditionally female attributes such as cooperation and caring.

You see this dichotomy immediately in health care where doctors were traditionally male and nurses traditionally female. Of course, this has been changing rapidly over the last few decades. The number of women in medical school in this country now outnumbers the number of men, although women are still unconsciously directed toward the more nurturing specialties such as primary care and psychiatry, and not toward the more technical surgical specialties.

The lack of social worth given to caregiving-type jobs is now making itself fully felt in this period of The Great Resignation with large numbers of the previously employed not returning to jobs that did not value them.

Every eldercare facility and company I'm aware of is short-staffed.

Wages are beginning to come up as employers desperately try to find and retain good employees, but it takes more than a decent paycheck to hold people in careers. It requires that their other social needs be met and that they feel that what they do is of value. When everything about their field is demeaned, why should they remain?

Someone once asked me what I thought the most important job category was in society that should be compensated on the highest salary scale. I thought about it for a moment and decided it was first-grade teachers.

These individuals instill in children a love of learning and inquiry that will ultimately lead to the absolute success of society in the long run. They determine literacy, the building blocks of math and science, and the basics of interpersonal relations with those who were previously strangers.

We all know, however, that elementary teachers aren't valued these days when teach-to-the-test is the mantra and they have the additional issues of political culture wars entering their classrooms.

I'm glad Mr. Rogers is dead. If he were still alive, I'm sure some conservative pundit would be decrying him from a spittle-flecked mouth for daring to embrace Critical Race Theory as he shares a wading pool with a man of another color.

This is one of those days when I wonder if our society is rapidly becoming irretrievably broken, just like one of my dining room chairs which splintered when I sat down in it this evening. (One of the minor annoyances of the day.) At least I have eleven others. I don't know that I'll ever have a sit-down dinner party for twelve again and, if I do, I guess one of the chairs won't match.

Another annoyance was having left my phone on the bed when I went off to work this morning. All sorts of things now run through my phone. It functions as my beeper. It's necessary for me to be able to sign prescriptions for controlled substances as the law dictates two separate authentications for the electronic health record. It's how I stay in touch with the VA when I'm at UAB and vice versa.

Funny how something that didn't exist a couple of decades ago has become so integrated into every aspect of our lives. I can tell that its presence is rewiring my brain as I felt lost this morning without it.

>———◁

On the positive side of the column, I sat last night with fellow actors and had a table read of *The Reindeer Monologues* which I'm performing in a few weeks, presuming I can stuff a nine-minute monologue into my rapidly aging brain. I hadn't been able to do something so mundane and as necessary as that for nearly two years, and it just felt good to be in that sort of space, making the sort of jokes theater people make when they're getting together and feeling each other out.

It's an eclectic cast—a couple of people I've worked with before, a couple of people I've known for years but never worked with, and a couple of people who are new to the game. It should be fun.

It's a small cast and crew, and most of our rehearsing will be individual, so I don't feel at all concerned about COVID safety. It passes the car test. I feel the chances of being injured or hurt in a car accident are higher than getting sick from working on this project.

Another positive is a reasonable raise at work. More money to donate to help keep theater in Birmingham afloat. I'll take some of it for a trip next year, but I haven't figured out when and where that will be.

Most of the extra projects are out of the way so I can concentrate on learning my monologue and enjoy a few days off in Seattle. The one last thing on the To-Do list is to write a sermon for church which I am delivering on Sunday the 5th.

I have entitled it *Book Writing and Other Happy Accidents*. It's going to cover some of the weird ways serendipity has impacted my life over the years.

The last time I gave a sermon (on issues surrounding gay marriage), it ended up getting published. Who knows what will happen with this one. Perhaps it will become a prologue.

In the meantime, it's off to bed, then up in the morning for VA house calls—complete with mask, hand sanitizer, and appropriate distancing.

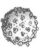

TUESDAY | NOVEMBER 23, 2021

THE PIECES DO NOT FIT. The center does not hold. And I imagine I am not alone in this feeling of existential malaise.

In the last month, the spread of COVID in Alabama has greatly abated. Positive tests, transmission numbers, hospitalizations—all down at levels not seen since last spring when vaccines had become plentiful and the Delta variant had not yet become established. Our case rate is less than 10 per 100,000, a benchmark that the WHO and the CDC use in determining if a pandemic is under control.

There are only about 400 people hospitalized state-wide, way down from the thousands a couple of months ago. But we are still losing about 13 Alabamians a day, which in my mind is 13 too many.

Does this mean the pandemic is over? I doubt it.

We're likely to see another surge or two in the next six months but, with luck, we'll see life continuing to normalize through 2022. The next big test is this coming holiday weekend and what this might mean for transmission chains as people gather. We'll learn that in mid-December as the inevitable changes in cases correspond to changes in behavior, only about two to three weeks later.

Where we go from here depends on three big and unknowable factors.

The first is the behavior of host organisms, mainly us humans (but being joined by various felines and white-tailed deer among others). Viruses do not book tickets for Thanksgiving or gather together in a crowded concert hall. People do, and viruses come along for the ride.

We're seeing a widely uneven distribution of cases at the moment. Here in the Deep South, we're having a bit of a breather, but Michigan and Minnesota are overrun with hospitals buckling under demand again. I strongly suspect colder temperatures and more time indoors among others may be the culprit, but I have no absolute data to back that up.

We're having the first freeze of the season tonight and cold temperatures for the rest of the week. If that has a bearing, we're going to see an increase based on this and Thanksgiving in December. Human behavior—which is not universally distributed—is our first unknowable variable. Some subpopulations continue to be cautious and mask. Some do not. Some are vaccinating their children which will interrupt transmission in classrooms and schoolyards. Some are not.

The second is what happens with the virus itself. It's constantly mutating. Most of those mutations are failures but a few are wildly successful like Delta which became the dominant strain within weeks in every geographic area in which it was introduced. It was that much more efficient at transmission and it had the unfortunate effect of also making certain middle-aged adults much more ill than the original strain, especially if they were unvaccinated.

We could get a mutation that makes the virus more infectious, one that makes it more deadly, or we may get lucky and get one that makes it less pathogenic. I still remain very worried about the issues with Long COVID and the possibilities of significant pathology that won't become apparent for years or even decades after infection, like post-polio syndrome in healthy adults who had and recovered from polio as children. Unlike the Mickey Mouse Club, every day is Anything Can Happen Day.

The third is the success of our treatments that may affect overall mortality curves going forward. We're at 773,000 deaths so far and the death rate nationwide remains fairly constant at just over 1,000 a day, so we're on track to be well over 800,000 by the new year. The distribution of those deaths keeps changing depending on where the hot spots are and the physiologic condition of victims.

In younger adults, where willful anti-vaccination ideas continue to run rampant, deaths are coming among healthy unvaccinated individuals. In the elderly, where vaccination is approaching universal (99% of Americans over 65 have at least one shot; over 85% are fully vaccinated), deaths are happening in vaccinated individuals, but mainly in those with significant immune or physiologic compromise at baseline, much as with influenza.

The introduction of the new oral antivirals may also change the trajectory as they are easy to distribute and for individuals to take, unlike the previous monoclonal antibody which required infusions in a clinic or hospital equipped for that procedure. Of course, they work early in the course of the disease. Those who engage in extreme COVID denialism stay home for weeks getting sicker and sicker—and only end up in the hospital when dragged there by family at death's door—aren't going to benefit much from them. Nor will they benefit much from ivermectin. Their bodies are too damaged at that point for easy repair.

≻━⊂

Back to my angst.

As things have been returning to normal locally, life patterns are also returning to normal and I, in my naiveté, am attempting to return to the activity levels I had in the fall of 2019 and winter of 2020 prior to the great pause.

I've been going to the theater (masked). I've been taking some classes in performance. I'm teaching Sunday school. I've had all of my usual work activities, and I've accepted a role that requires me to learn a nine-minute monologue (off-book date is December 1).

This was my usual load of activities not so long ago and I had no trouble keeping the balls in the air. Now, however, I feel like I'm failing.

I always feel one step behind. Maybe it's the fact that I added a third career over the course of the pandemic which has its own set of obligations and worries, and there's now too much on my plate, but I think it's something deeper than this. I think I'm a fundamentally different person than I was the second week of March 2020. Too much has happened.

My brain has been rewired by living in an environment of constant danger, a new one for most of us and, as we emerge from our pandemic lives, we're all going to find that certain things just feel wrong and that the pieces just don't fit the way we think they should.

I think we're all going to have to be gentle with each other over the next couple of years, and we're going to have to encourage our society, our workplaces, our schools, and all of our other institutions to understand this.

It's going to be tough.

The business of America is business and the purpose of business is to make as much money as possible. Trying to steer away from this to something that puts human capital ahead of financial capital is going to be very difficult, but I think it's going to be necessary. If we don't, we're going to see a number of sectors of our economy crater.

The service sector is in trouble due to people having resigned from low-level jobs after figuring out new ways of living. The health-care system is headed for a major crash due to the confluence of experienced employees leaving their jobs due to the incredible stresses of the last few years and the enormous increase in demand that is just beginning to happen with the aging of the Baby Boom.

Education is in trouble. The ill-preparedness of the American education system for pandemic schooling has left children behind developmentally and with more significant behavior problems cropping up in schools. Parent behavior isn't much better, and a raft of experienced teachers is rapidly heading for the exits due to the stresses of the last two years and the rising levels of abuse that administrators seem reluctant to quell.

All of this uncertainty is, of course, fanning the flames of authoritarianism in the political system as people, feeling unmoored and abnormal, turn to those who promise certainties and rules and a return to a past that never actually existed.

None of this is unique to the United States.

Eastern European states such as Poland and Hungary have redone their political systems in full authoritarian and illiberal patterns. In Western Europe, just as here, there are right-wing authoritarian movements piggybacking on mistakes in coronavirus response. The Dutch police were out on the streets of Rotterdam with water cannons routing anti-vax protestors, and in Austria, the government is handling their anti-vax minority by locking down again and making it practically impossible to function without vaccine documentation.

Will we go the way of Orban in Hungary or Bolsonaro in Brazil or Erdogan in Turkey? It's hard to say.

The conservative wing of the Republican party has gone all-in for this thinking (CPAC is even scheduled for Budapest next year rather than Washington DC) and, as the party continues to purge moderates or more independent thinkers, we will continue heading there if we elect a Republican congress and executive in the next few years.

The Democrats are countering by trying to show the American people that big government and big ideas can help individual Americans. We have the infrastructure bill. We'll find out shortly if we get the Build Back Better bill.

The problem with the Democrats is that they have a very poor track record of messaging in terms the American public can easily understand. The Republicans use Fox and all of their websites and pundits to deliver a clear and unified message that is easily digested by their followers. The Democrats do not. And the mainstream media is so involved in making sure there's an exciting horse race between red and blue that we're lucky we get any real news out of them at all.

><>

I couldn't sleep tonight so I spent my time writing all of this.

Fortunately, due to the short week with the holiday, I don't have that much to do at work tomorrow. If I am dragging around a bit, I'll likely be forgiven. I'll have several large cups of coffee and that should keep me going.

Now I'm going to flip on Netflix, not to watch *Tick Tick Boom* as I need to have full mental faculties for that, but to finish up *Midnight Mass*, Mike Flanagan's latest supernatural/horror limited series. I started watching them with *The Haunting of Hill House* which I tuned into initially as I had friends on the production crew, and I try to support my friends and their artistic endeavors.

The first few episodes of *Midnight Mass* felt like a moody psychological drama and then, about a third of the way in, there was an abrupt shift in plot and tone to Stephen King Land with more than a few echoes of 'Salems Lot.

I was going to give up on it at that point, but kept watching and, as it went on, I realized that the point of the series was not the monster movie or the horror drama. The series is a very clever allegory on the function of religion and how, when religion becomes fundamentalist and overly structured regarding creed and belief, it becomes easy for the followers to become seduced, in the name of religion, away from good to evil without understanding that their hard lines of us versus them are creating monstrous outcomes.

It doesn't take too long to think of dozens of examples of conservative sects of all faiths where this is currently happening. And it's getting worse, dovetailing with the political issues I noted above.

I can't fix politics. I can't fix religion. I can't fix coronavirus. I'm not even sure I can fix my own life.

What I am sure of is that it's Thanksgiving week. I'm heading to Seattle to be with my family. It's one of the few bulwarks I have against the existential problems besieging all of us these days. Time to rejuvenate and to leave a crumbling health system, political strife, and news articles about a new variant, named Omicron by WHO, which seems to be emerging in South Africa.

While in Seattle, I can keep abreast of local transmission. Wear my mask indoors in crowds, keep my hands washed, not get in other people's personal space, and try to maintain good health habits.

I think that will do for now.

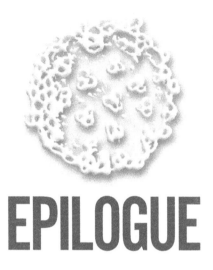

EPILOGUE

Ev'ry Time We Say Goodbye

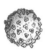

SUNDAY | SEPTEMBER 18, 2022

'VE SPENT THE LAST SIX WEEKS finalizing these entries in *The Accidental Plague Diaries* into book form. It's been an interesting experience, going back over the last eighteen months or so. It's been a sobering reminder of how fast the pandemic is changing the world around us in a myriad of ways. The Delta variant and the politics around the original vaccine rollout almost seem like historical artifacts of decades ago, not recent events, overshadowed as they have been by the rise of Omicron, newer boosters, and the surges that seem to come with uncomfortable regularity.

From where we sit this fall, the pandemic is improving but is still not over. We continue to lose hundreds of American lives daily. We have no idea what new mutations may be coming. Masking and other good habits have more or less fallen by the wayside as we struggle to get back to pre-pandemic modes of living, an impossible task as we are no longer the same people we were in early 2020.

I think that's the biggest challenge that currently faces us as a people, not just here in the USA but worldwide. We can't go back to before, we must go forward into new patterns dictated by the people we have lost, the lessons we have learned, the institutions we have both inadvertently and deliberately damaged.

How do we do that? I don't know. But I'll continue to observe and record and, with time and good fortune, eventually end these writings on a hopeful note as we all move together into the unknown future. For that's all we've ever been able to do.

ABOUT THE AUTHOR

ANDREW DUXBURY is originally from Seattle, Washington. He received his BS in chemistry and biology from Stanford University and his MD from the University of Washington.

He spent his early career at UC Davis in Sacramento where he discovered the fascinating world of geriatric medicine and his first husband, Steve Spivey. He later left the West Coast for the Deep South and the geriatrics faculty of the University of Alabama at Birmingham where he continues to teach and practice geriatric medicine.

After the untimely death of his first husband, shortly after moving to Alabama, he decided to rebalance his life, beginning a second career as a performer and picking up a second husband, Tommy Thompson, along the way.

Tommy also died young, leading to additional introspection and a third career as a writer. Dr. Duxbury continues to muddle through life in Birmingham with his two cats, Oliver and Binx, a host of friends, and his trusty laptop.

CPSIA information can be obtained
at www.ICGtesting.com
Printed in the USA
JSHW050856171122
33329JS00004B/10